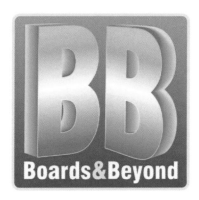

Boards and Beyond:
Endocrinology Slides

Slides from the Boards and Beyond Website

Jason Ryan, MD, MPH

2019 Edition

Table of Contents

Thyroid Gland

Jason Ryan, MD, MPH

Thyroid Anatomy

- Two lobes (left, right)
- Isthmus: thin band of tissue between lobes
- Sometimes pyramidal lobe above isthmus

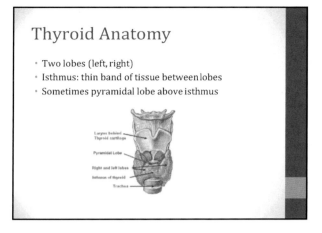

Thyroid Anatomy

- Blood supply: superior and inferior thyroid arteries
- Superior thyroid: 1st branch external carotid artery
- Inferior thyroid: Thyrocervical trunk (off subclavian)

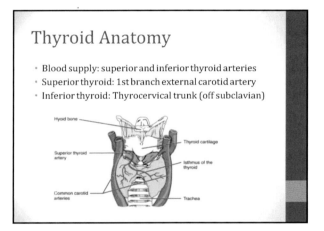

Thyroid Embryology

- Forms from floor of pharynx (epithelial cells)

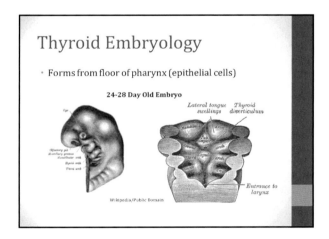

24-28 Day Old Embryo

Wikipedia/Public Domain

Thyroid Embryology

- Descends into neck
- Initially maintains connection to tongue
  - Thyroglossal duct
  - Disappears later in development
- Two remnants of duct in child/adult
  - Foramen cecum in tongue
  - Pyramidal lobe of thyroid

Foramen Cecum

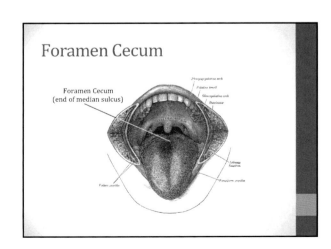

Foramen Cecum
(end of median sulcus)

Thyroglossal Duct Cyst

- Persistent remnant of thyroglossal duct
- **Midline neck mass; usually painless**
- Usually discovered in childhood
- Classically, move up with swallowing or tongue protrusion
- May contain thyroid cells

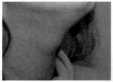

Klaus D. Peter, Gummersbach, Germany

Ectopic Thyroid

- Functioning thyroid tissue outside of gland
- Most common location is **base of tongue**
- Presents as a mass in the tongue
  - Commonly detected during increased demand for hormones
  - Puberty and pregnancy
- May be the only functioning thyroid tissue
  - May under-produce thyroid hormone → **hypothyroidism**
  - ↑ TSH → growth of ectopic tissue

Thyroid Histology

- Thyroid gland contains "follicles"
- Filled with colloid (protein material)
- Single layer of epithelial cells lines each follicle
  - "Follicular cells"
- Hormone synthesized by follicular cells

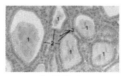

Uwe Gille/Wikipedia

Thyroid Hormones

- Contain the element **iodine**
- **Iodized salt**
  - Table salt (NaCl) mixed with small minute amount of iodine
  - Done in many countries to prevent iodine deficiency
  - Added to salt in US in 1924

Thyroid Hormones

- Two hormones: T3 and T4
- Synthesized from tyrosine and iodine

Tyrosine

Triiodothyronine (T₃)   Thyroxine (T₄)

Thyroglobulin

- Large protein
- Produced by thyroid follicular cells
- Contains numerous tyrosine molecules

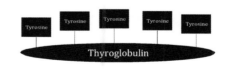

Iodine

- **Iodine** = I (chemical element, atomic number 53)
- **Iodide** = iodine bound to another atom
  - "Iodide salt" with negative charge (I⁻)
  - Potassium iodide = KI
  - Plasma iodine exists as iodide salt
- For thyroid hormone, iodide in our diet needs to be:
  - Taken up by follicular cells
  - Oxidized to I_2 (undergo "**oxidation**")
  - Added to organic/carbon structures ("**organification**")

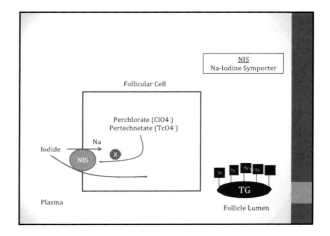

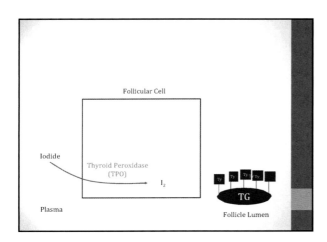

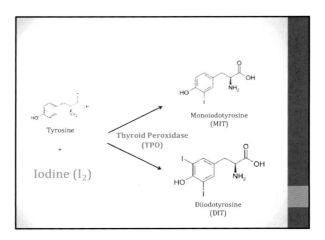

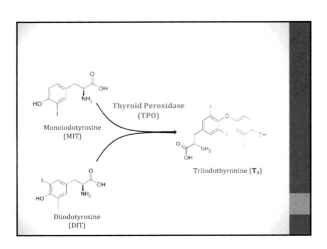

Hormone Synthesis
Coupling Reactions

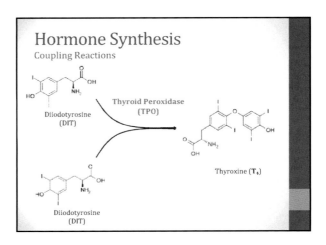

TPO
Thyroid Peroxidase

- Multifunctional enzyme
- Catalyzes:
  - Oxidation of iodide
  - Organification of iodine into MIT/DIT
  - Coupling of MIT/DIT into T3/T4
- TPO antibodies common in autoimmune thyroid disease

Hormone Synthesis

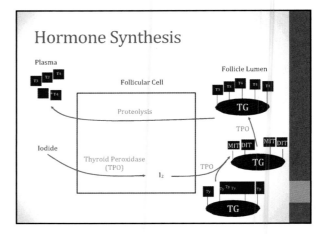

Thyroid Hormones

- T4 is major hormone produced by thyroid gland
  - >90% of thyroid hormone produced is T4
- T3 more potent hormone
- T4 is a "prohormone" for T3
- 5' deiodinase converts T4 → T3
- Most conversion occurs in **peripheral tissues**

Thyroxine (T_4) — 5'-deiodinase → Triiodothyronine (T_3)

Hyperthyroid Medications

- **Propylthiouracil (PTU)**
  - Inhibits TPO: ↓ T3/T4 from thyroid gland
  - Inhibits 5'-deiodinase: ↓ T4 to T3 conversion peripherally
- **Methimazole**
  - Inhibits TPO

  > PTU and Methimazole are both "thioamides"

- **Propranolol**
  - Beta blocker
  - Weak inhibitor of 5'-deiodinase
  - Excellent drug in thyrotoxicosis
  - Blocks catecholamines and T4-T3 conversion

Wolff-Chaikoff Effect

- Excessive iodide in diet could lead to hyperthyroidism
- Thyroid protects itself via **Wolff-Chaikoff Effect**
- **Organification** inhibited by ↑ iodide
  - Less synthesis of MIT/DIT

Amiodarone

- Class III antiarrhythmic drug
- Commonly used in atrial fibrillation
- Contains iodine
- Can cause **hypothyroidism** via excess iodine
  - Wolff-Chaikoff Effect

Amiodarone

- Mimics T4
  - Inhibits 5'-deiodinase
  - ↓T3 → ↑TSH from pituitary gland
  - TSH rises after start of therapy then normalizes

Radioactive Iodine

- I^{131} is an isotope of iodine
  - Has 53 protons like elemental iodine
  - Extra neutrons
- Emits radiation (β-decay)
- Exposure → radioactive iodine in thyroid gland
  - Competes with elemental iodine for uptake
  - Will concentrate in thyroid gland
- Small dose: Used for imaging
- Large dose: Destroys thyroid tissue
  - Used as therapy for hyperthyroidism

TBG
Thyroxine-Binding Globulin

- Most plasma thyroid hormone is T4
- Thyroid hormones poorly soluble in water
- Most T4 is bound to TBG
  - Some with transthyretin and albumin
  - TBG present in small amount but has high affinity
  - TBG produced in liver
- Key point:
  - Less TBG → less available T4/T3 to tissues

TBG-T4 → T4

TBG
Thyroxine-Binding Globulin

- **Estrogen** raises TBG levels
  - Modifies TBG molecules
  - Slows clearance from plasma
  - **Pregnancy, OCP users**
  - Will raise total T4 levels
- **Liver failure** lowers TBG levels
  - Less production of protein
  - Can lower total T4 levels

TBG
Thyroxine-Binding Globulin

Rise in TBG
↓
More bound T4
↓
Less free T4
↓
↑TSH
↓
↑Total T4
↓
↑ Free T4 (back to normal)
↓
↓TSH (back to normal)

Thyroid Hormone Receptor

- Family of nuclear receptors
- Hormone-activated transcription factors
- Modulate gene expression

Effects of Thyroid Hormone

- Major regulator of **metabolic activity** and **growth**
- Glucose, lipid metabolism
- Cardiac function
- Bone growth
- CNS development

Thyroid Hormone
Metabolic Effects

- ↑ Carbohydrate Metabolism
  - ↑ glycogenolysis, gluconeogenesis
- ↑ Fat Metabolism
  - ↑ lipolysis
  - ↓ concentrations of cholesterol, triglycerides
  - ↑ low-density lipoprotein receptors in liver (↓ LDL)
  - ↑ cholesterol secretion in bile
- Hypothyroid patients: ↑ **cholesterol**
- Hyperthyroid patients: **hyperglycemia**

Thyroid Hormone
Metabolic Effects

- ↑ basal metabolic rate
  - Basal rate of energy use per time
  - Amount of energy burned if you slept all day
- ↑ Na/K ATPase pumps
  - More pumps = more ATP consumed
  - ↑ oxygen demand to replenish ATP
  - ↑ respiratory rate
  - ↑ body temperature
- Hyperthyroid patients: **weight loss**

McDonough AA, et al. **Thyroid hormone coordinately regulates Na+-K+-ATPase alpha- and beta-subunit mRNA levels in kidney.** Am J Physiol. 1988 Feb;254(2 Pt 1):C323-9.

Thyroid Hormone
Cardiac Effects

- ↑ CO/HR/SV/contractility
- ↑ β1 receptors in heart
- Hyperthyroid patients: **Tachycardia**

Thyroid Hormone
CNS and Bone effects

- TH required for normal bone growth/CNS maturation
- Childhood hypothyroidism → **cretinism**
  - Stunted growth
  - Mental retardation
- Causes
  - Iodine deficiency (3rd world)
  - Thyroid dysgenesis
  - Inborn errors of hormone synthesis (dyshormonogenesis)
  - TPO most common

Thyroid Hormone
CNS and Bone effects

- Most common **treatable** cause of mental retardation
- Most babies appear normal
  - Maternal T3/T4 crosses placenta
- Newborn screening programs
  - Measure T4 or TSH from heel-stick blood specimens

Thyroid Hormone
CNS and Bone effects

- Mental retardation
- Coarse facial features
- Short stature
- Umbilical hernia
- Enlarged tongue

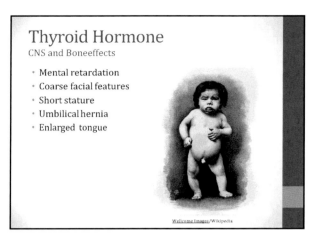

Wellcome Images/Wikipedia

Thyroid Hormone Regulation

- **TSH (thyrotropin)** released by anterior pituitary
- Binds to receptors on follicular cells
- Activates cAMP/PKA 2nd messenger system
- ↑ T3/T4 release
  - ↑ rate of proteolysis of thyroglobulin
  - Leads to rapid release of more T3/T4
  - Also stimulates thyroid cell growth, TG synthesis

Thyroid Hormone Regulation

- Serum T4/T3 level sensed by hypothalamus
- Releases thyroid releasing hormone (TRH)

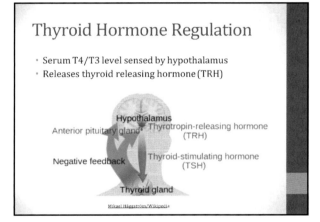

Mikael Häggström/Wikipedia

Pregnancy

- Multiple effects on thyroid hormone production
  - Rise in total plasma T4/T3 levels
  - Rise in TBG levels (estrogen)
- hCG stimulates thyroid (same alpha unit as TSH)
- Raises free T4 → lower TSH

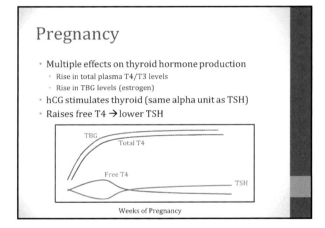

Thyroid Panel

- Four standard measurements to assess thyroid

Test	Normal Value
TSH	0.4 to 5.0 mU/L
Total T4	60 to 145 nmol/L
Total T3	1.1 to 3 nmol/L
Free T4	0.01-0.03 nmol/L

Note:
T4 > T3
Total T4 >> Free T4
(most bound to TBG)

Calcitonin

- Hormone produced by thyroid
- Synthesized by **parafollicular cells** (C-cells)

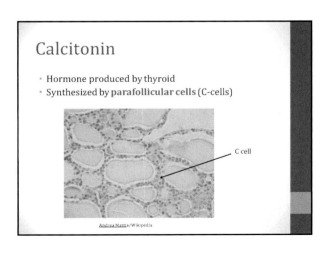

Andrea Mazza/Wikipedia

Calcitonin

- Lowers serum **calcium**
  - Suppresses resorption of bone; inhibits osteoclasts
  - Inhibits renal reabsorption of calcium, phosphorus
  - Increased calcium in urine
- Probably minor role in calcium handling in humans
- Used as pharmacologic therapy for **hypercalcemia**

Thyroid Disorders

Jason Ryan, MD, MPH

Thyroid Disorders

Thyroid Disorders

Hyperthyroid   Hypothyroid   Thyroiditis

Hypothyroidism

- Metabolism **SLOWS DOWN**
- Lethargy, fatigue
- Weakness; dyspnea on exertion
- Cold intolerance
- Weight gain with loss of appetite
- Constipation
- Hyporeflexia
- Dry, cool skin
- Coarse, brittle hair
- Bradycardia

Hyperlipidemia

- Classic feature of hypothyroidism
- ↑ total cholesterol
- ↑ LDL cholesterol
- Primary mechanism: ↓ **LDL receptor density**
  - T_3 upregulates LDL receptor gene activation

Myxedema
Thyroid dermopathy

- **Non-pitting** edema of the skin from hypothyroidism
- Hyaluronic acid deposits in dermis
- Draws water out → swelling
- Usually facial/periorbital swelling
- Pretibial myxedema
  - Special form of myxedema over shin
  - Seen in Grave's disease (hyperthyroidism)
- Myxedema coma = coma from hypothyroidism

Myxedema
Thyroid dermopathy

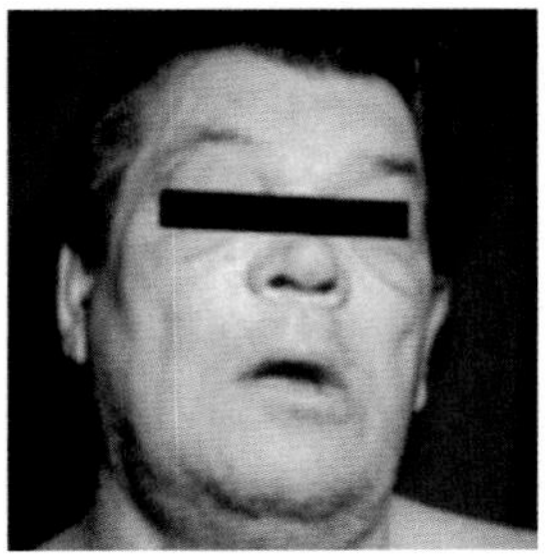

Herbert L. Fred, MD and Hendrik A. van Dijk

Hypothyroid Myopathy

- Muscle symptoms common in hypothyroid
- Weakness, cramps, myalgias
- ↑ serum **creatine kinase (CK)** common (up to 90%)

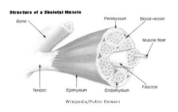

Wikipedia/Public Domain

Hyponatremia

- Hypothyroidism is a well-described cause ↓Na
- High levels of ADH (SIADH)
- May lead to confusion

Thyroid Replacement

- Levothyroxine (Synthroid): synthetic T4
- Liothyronine (Cytomel): synthetic T3
- Levothyroxine preferred
  - T3 absorbed from intestines rapidly
  - Can cause mild **hyperthyroidism symptoms**
  - Tachycardia, tremor
  - Also, T4 converted to T3
- Titrate dose until **TSH is normal**

Hyperthyroidism

- Metabolism **SPEEDS UP**
- Hyperactivity
- Heat intolerance
- Weight loss with increased appetite
- Diarrhea
- Hyperreflexia
- Warm, moist skin
- Fine hair
- Tachycardia (atrial fibrillation)

Thyroid Storm

- Life-threatening hyperthyroidism (thyrotoxicosis)
- Usually precipitated by acute event
  - Patient with pre-existing hyperthyroid disease
  - Grave's or toxic multinodular goiter
  - Surgery, trauma, infection
- Massive **catecholamine** surge
- Fever, delirium
- Tachycardia with **death from arrhythmia**
- Hyperglycemia (catecholamines/thyroid hormone)
- Hypercalcemia (bone turnover)

Goiter

- Enlarged thyroid
- High TSH, inability to produce T3/T4
- Thyroid stimulating antibodies (Grave's)

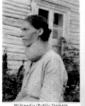

Wikipedia/Public Domain

Lab Findings

- Best initial test is TSH

TSH

Lab Findings

- Most disorders are primary disease
  - Disorder of the thyroid gland
  - TSH is opposite thyroid hormone
  - Hypothyroidism = ↑ TSH with low T3/T4
  - Hyperthyroidism = ↓ TSH with high T3/T4

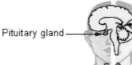

Pituitary gland

Thyroid gland

Lab Findings

- Central hyper/hypo thyroid disease
  - Low TSH and low T3/T4; High TSH and high T3/T4
  - Rare disorders of the pituitary, hypothalamus
  - Usually hypothalamic-pituitary tumors
  - Tumors block secretion TRH/TSH (hypothyroidism)
  - Rarely a TSHoma can secrete TSH (hyperthyroidism)
  - Pituitary resistance to thyroid hormone (hyperthyroidism)

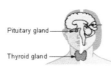

Pituitary gland

Thyroid gland

Reverse T3

- Isomer of T3 also derived from T4

HO

Revere T3

Thyroxine (T₄)

Triiodothyronine (T₃)

Reverse T3

- Level usually parallels T4
  - Low T4 → Low rT3
- One special use: **Euthyroid sick syndrome**
  - Critically ill patients → low TSH → Low T3/T4
  - Can look like central hypothyroidism
  - rT3 rises in critical illness (impaired clearance)
- Critically ill patient with low TSH/T4/T3
  - Check rT3
  - Low → central hypothyroidism
  - High → sick euthyroid syndrome

Hyperthyroidism

- **Grave's disease (#1 cause)**
- Toxic multinodular goiter
- Amiodarone
- Iodine load
- Early thyroiditis

Grave's Disease

- Autoimmune disease
- Thyroid stimulating antibodies produced
- Symptoms of hyperthyroidism occur

Grave's Disease

- Exophthalmos (bulging eyes)
  - Proptosis (protrusion of eye) and periorbital edema
  - Usually no ocular symptoms
- Pretibial myxedema (shins)
- T-cell lymphocyte activation of fibroblasts
- Fibroblasts contain TSH receptor
- Stimulation → secretion of glycosaminoglycans
  - Hydrophilic substances, mostly hyaluronic acid
  - Draws in water → swelling

Grave's Disease

Jonathan Trobe, M.D./Wikipedia

Herbert L. Fred, MD and Hendrik A. van Dijk

Grave's Disease

- Diagnosis:
  - Usually hyperthyroid labs plus exophthalmos
  - Can measure TSH receptor antibodies
  - "Thyroid stimulating immunoglobulins"
- Treatment
  - Symptoms: beta blockers, thionamides
  - Drugs often started in preparation for definitive therapy
  - Radioactive iodine ablation or surgery

Thionamides

- Methimazole
  - Inhibits thyroid peroxidase (TPO)
  - Organification of iodine
  - Coupling of MIT/DIT
- Propylthiouracil (PTU)
  - Inhibits TPO
  - Also inhibits 5'-deiodinase
  - Blunts peripheral conversion T4→T3

Thionamides

- Skin rash (common)
- Agranulocytosis
  - Rare drop in WBC
  - May present as fever, infection after starting drug
  - WBC improves with stopping drug
  - Aplastic anemia cases reported
- Hepatotoxicity

Thionamides

- Methimazole: teratogen
  - Associated with congenital malformations
  - Especially 1st trimester
  - PTU often used during early pregnancy

Thyroid Storm
Treatment

- Propranolol
  - Beta blocker
  - Blocks T4 → T3 conversion
- Thionamides (PTU, Methimazole)
- SSKI (saturated solution of potassium iodide)
  - Iodide load → shuts down T4 production
  - Wolff-Chaikoff effect
- Steroids
  - Reduce T4 → T3 conversion
  - Suppress auto-immune damage
  - Treat possible concomitant adrenal insufficiency

Grave's Ophthalmopathy

- Sometimes worsens despite treating hyperthyroidism
- Can cause irritation, excessive tearing , pain
- Symptoms often worse by cold air, wind, bright lights
- Severe inflammation treatments:
  - Steroids
  - Radiation
  - Surgery

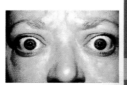

Jonathan Trobe, M.D /Wikipedia

Toxic Adenomas

- Nodules in thyroid that function independently
  - Usually contain mutated TSH receptor
  - Do not respond to TSH
  - One nodule: Toxic adenoma
  - Multiple: Toxic multinodular goiter
- Findings:
  - Palpable nodule
  - Hyperthyroidism symptoms/labs
- Treatment: Radioactive iodine or surgery

Radioactive Iodine Uptake

- Important test for thyroid nodules
- Administration of I^{131} (lower dose than ablation)
- Contraindicated in pregnancy/breastfeeding
- "Hot" nodule
  - Takes up I^{131}
  - Not-cancerous
- "Cold" nodule
  - Chance of cancer (~5%)
  - Often biopsied (Fine-needle aspiration)

Jod-Basedow Phenomenon

- **Iodine-induced hyperthyroidism**
- Often occurs in regions of **iodine deficiency**
  - Introduction of iodine → hyperthyroidism
- Often occurs in patients with **toxic adenomas**
  - Drugs administered with high iodine content
  - Expectorants (potassium iodide)
  - CT contrast dye
  - Amiodarone

Amiodarone

- Two types of hyperthyroidism
- Type I
  - Occurs in patients with **pre-existing thyroid disease**
  - Grave's or Multi-nodular goiter
  - Amiodarone provides iodine → excess hormone production
- Type II
  - Destructive thyroiditis
  - Excess release T4/ T3 (no ↑ hormone synthesis)
  - Direct toxic effect of drug
  - Can occur in patients without pre-existing thyroid illness

Hypothyroidism

- Iodine deficiency
- Iodine excess
- Congenital hypothyroidism
- Amiodarone
- Thyroiditis
  - Hashimoto's (#1 cause when dietary iodine is sufficient)
  - Subacute
  - Riedel's

Iodine Deficiency

- "Endemic goiter"
  - Goiter in region with widespread iodine deficiency
  - Common in mountainous areas (iodine depleted by run-off)
- Constant elevation of TSH → enlarged thyroid

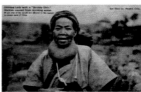

Wellcome Images

Iodine Excess

- Excessive iodide in diet could lead to hyperthyroidism
- Thyroid protects itself via **Wolff-Chaikoff Effect**
- **Organification** inhibited by ↑ iodide
  - Less synthesis of MIT/DIT
- Chronic, high iodine intake → goiter/hypothyroidism

Iodine

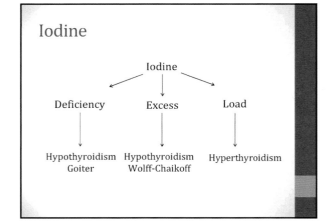

Goitrogens

- Substances that inhibit thyroid hormone production
- Most common is iodine
- **Lithium** (inhibits release of thyroid hormone)
- Certain foods (cassava and millet)

Amiodarone

- Can cause **hypothyroidism**
- Excess iodine → Wolff-Chaikoff Effect
  - Suppression of thyroid hormone synthesis
  - Normal patients "escape" in few weeks
  - Pre-existing subclinical thyroid disease → "failure to escape"
- Also mimics T4
  - Inhibits 5'-diodinase

Amiodarone

Always check TSH before starting amiodarone

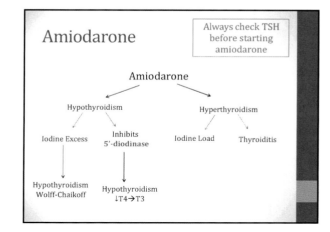

Congenital Hypothyroidism

- TH required for normal bone growth/CNS maturation
- Childhood hypothyroidism → **cretinism**
  - Stunted growth
  - Mental retardation
- Causes
  - Iodine deficiency (3rd world)
  - Thyroid dysgenesis
  - Inborn errors of hormone synthesis (dyshormonogenesis)
  - TPO most common

Thyroid Hormone
CNS and Bone effects

- Most common **treatable** cause of mental retardation
- Newborn screening programs
  - Measure T4 or TSH from heel-stick blood specimens

Thyroid Hormone
CNS and Bone effects

- Mental retardation
- Coarse facial features
- Short stature
- Umbilical hernia
- Enlarged tongue

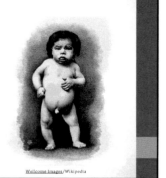

Wellcome Images/Wikipedia

Iatrogenic Hypothyroidism

- Thyroid surgery
  - Often done for Grave's or malignancy
- Radioiodine therapy
  - I^{131} administered orally as solution or capsule
  - Beta-emissions → tissue damage
  - Ablation of thyroid function over weeks
  - Done for Grave's or malignancy
- Neck radiation
  - Hodgkin's lymphoma
  - Head and neck cancer

Hashimoto's Thyroiditis
Chronic Autoimmune Thyroiditis

- Most common cause of hypothyroidism (non-diet)
- **Lymphocytes** infiltrate thyroid gland
  - Autoimmune disorder (T-cell attack thyroid; B cell activation)
  - HLA-DR5

Hashimoto's Thyroiditis
Chronic Autoimmune Thyroiditis

- Antibodies produced
  - Anti-TPO
  - Anti-thyroglobulin
- Histology:
  - Massive lymphocytic infiltrate (germinal centers)
  - Hurthle cells (enlarged eosinophilic follicular cells)

Hashimoto's Thyroiditis
Chronic Autoimmune Thyroiditis

- Primarily occurs in women
- Enlarged non-tender thyroid gland
- Gradual loss of thyroid function → symptoms
- Symptoms/labs of hypothyroidism
- Treatment: thyroid hormone replacement
- Increased risk of Non Hodgkin B cell lymphoma

Subacute Thyroiditis
de Quervain's/granulomatous thyroiditis

- **Granulomatous** inflammation of thyroid
- Occurs in young females
- **Tender**, enlarged thyroid gland
- Hyperthyroid → euthyroid → hypothyroid
- Treatment:
  - Anti-inflammatories (aspirin, NSAIDs, steroids)
  - Thyroid symptoms usually mild (no treatment)
  - Usually resolves in few weeks

Riedel's Thyroiditis

- Fibroblast activation/proliferation
- **Fibrous tissue** (collagen) deposition in thyroid
- "Rock hard" thyroid
- Often extends **beyond the thyroid**
  - Parathyroid glands → hypoparathyroidism
  - Recurrent laryngeal nerves → hoarseness
  - Trachea compression → difficulty breathing
- Associated with **IgG4 plasma cells**
  - May be an "IgG4-related disease" (autoimmune pancreatitis)
  - IgG4 plasma cells identified in biopsy specimens

Lymphocytic Thyroiditis
Painless Thyroiditis

- Variant of Hashimoto's
- Lymphocytic infiltration of thyroid gland
- Transient hyperthyroidism
  - Can look like Grave's without eye/skin findings
  - Serum thyroid stimulating immunoglobulins not elevated
- Followed sometimes by hypothyroidism
  - Can look like Hashimoto's
- Usually self-limited (weeks)

Thyroid Cancer

Jason Ryan, MD, MPH

General Principles

- Thyroid cancer usually no hyper/hypo symptoms
- Often presents as nodule
- Differential is benign adenoma versus cancer
- Biopsy done by **fine needle aspiration**

Thyroid Imaging

- **Ultrasound**
  - Some characteristics suggest cancer
  - Borders, vascularity, calcifications

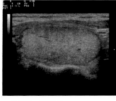

Nevit Dilmen/Wikipedia

Radioactive Iodine Uptake

- Small oral dose I^{131} given to patient
- Scintillation camera → image of thyroid
- Normal: diffuse, even uptake
- Diffuse high uptake: Grave's
- Diffuse low uptake: Hashimoto's
- Multiple areas of high uptake: nodular goiter
- Single "hot" nodule: adenoma
- Single "cold" nodule: Possible cancer
  - Most cancers do not make hormone
  - About 10% cold nodules are malignant

Myohan /Wikipedia

Follicular Adenoma

- Common cause of thyroid nodules
- Benign proliferation of follicles
- Normal follicular tissue seen on biopsy
- **Completely surrounded by fibrous capsule**
- **FNA cannot distinguish between adenomas/cancer**
  - Cannot see entire capsule
  - Follicular carcinoma has similar histology by FNA
- FNA follicular pathology followed over time
  - Growth, suspicious new findings → surgery

Thyroid Cancer

- Papillary
- Follicular
- Medullary
- Anaplastic

Papillary Carcinoma

- Most common form thyroid cancer (~80%)
- Increased risk with **prior radiation exposure**
  - Childhood chest radiation for mediastinal malignancy or acne
  - Survivors of atomic bomb detonation (Japan)
  - Nuclear power plant accidents (Chernobyl)
- Presents as thyroid nodule
  - Sometimes seen on chest/neck imaging (CT/MRI)
  - Diagnosis made after fine needle aspiration (FNA)
- Excellent prognosis
  - Treated with surgery plus radioactive iodine ablation

Papillary Carcinoma

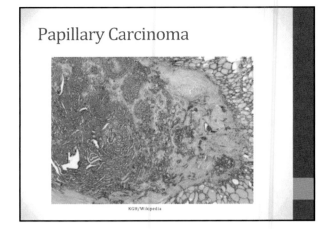

KGH/Wikipedia

Papillary Carcinoma

- Three key pathology findings:
  - Psammoma bodies
  - Nuclear grooves
  - Orphan Annie's Eye Nuclei
- Diagnosis made by **nuclear findings**

Psammoma Bodies

- Calcifications with an layered pattern
- Seen in other neoplasms but only papillary for thyroid

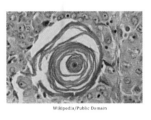

Wikipedia/Public Domain

Nuclear Grooves

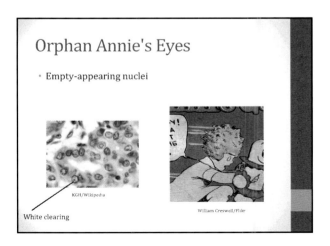

KGH/Wikipedia

Orphan Annie's Eyes

- Empty-appearing nuclei

KGH/Wikipedia

White clearing

William Creswell/Flikr

Follicular Carcinoma

- Similar to follicular adenoma
- Breaks through ("**invades**") fibrous capsule
- **FNA cannot distinguish between adenomas/cancer**
- Follicular pathology followed over time
  - Growth, suspicious new findings → surgery

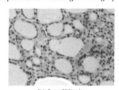

Yale Rosen/Wikipedia

Follicular Carcinoma

- Possible **hematogenous** metastasis
- Treatment:
  - Thyroidectomy
  - I^{131} to ablate any remaining tissue or metastasis

Medullary Carcinoma

- Cancer of parafollicular cells (C cells)
- Produces calcitonin
  - Lowers serum calcium
  - Normally minimal effect on calcium levels
  - With malignancy → **hypocalcemia**
- **Amyloid deposits in thyroid**
  - Amyloid = protein deposits
  - Calcitonin = peptide
  - Appearance of amyloid on biopsy

Medullary Carcinoma

Malignant cells/Amyloid "stroma"

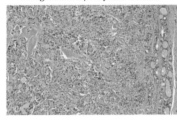

Nephron/Wikipedia

MEN Syndromes
Multiple Endocrine Neoplasia

- Gene mutations that run in families
- Cause multiple endocrine tumors
- MEN 2A and 2B associated with medullary carcinoma
  - Caused by RET oncogene mutation
  - Some patients have **elective thyroidectomy**

Anaplastic Carcinoma
Undifferentiated Carcinoma

- Occurs in **elderly**
- Highly malignant - invades local tissues
  - Dysphagia (esophagus)
  - Hoarseness (recurrent laryngeal nerve)
  - Dyspnea (trachea)
  - Don't confuse with Riedel's ("rock hard" thyroid/young pt)
- Poor prognosis
- Pathology: Undifferentiated cells
  - No papilla, follicles, or amyloid

Adrenal Glands

Jason Ryan, MD, MPH

Adrenal Glands

- Located above kidneys
- Arteries: Suprarenal arteries
  - Left and right
  - Superior, inferior, middle
- Veins:
  - Right adrenal → IVC

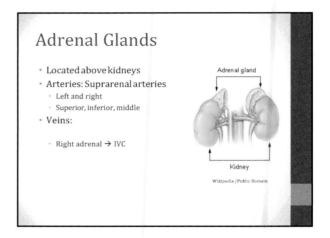

Wikipedia/Public Domain

Cortex and Medulla

- Cortex: Three groups of hormones
  - Mineralocorticoids (aldosterone)
  - Glucocorticoids (cortisol)
  - Androgens (testosterone)
  - Derived from **mesoderm**
- Medulla
  - Epinephrine and norepinephrine
  - Sympathetic nervous system control
  - Derived from neural crest

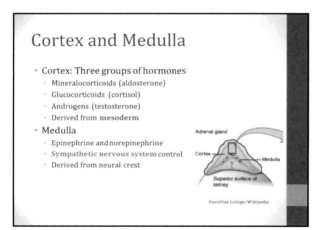

OpenStax College/Wikipedia

Signal Transmission

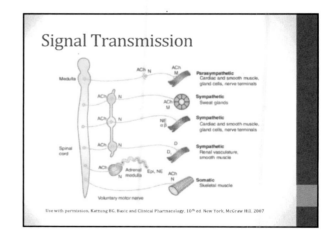

Use with permission. Katzung BG. Basic and Clinical Pharmacology. 10th ed. New York, McGraw Hill, 2007

Mineralocorticoids

- Most important is **aldosterone**
- Key effects on kidney function
- Release controlled by RAA system
  - **Renin-angiotensin-aldosterone**
- Increase Na^+/Water resorption
- Promote K^+/H^+ excretion

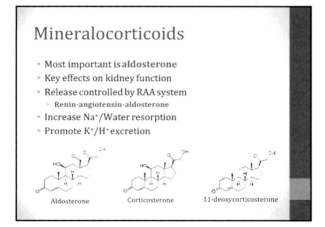

Aldosterone   Corticosterone   11-deoxycorticosterone

Collecting Duct

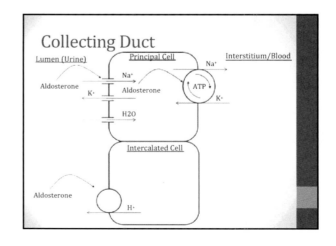

Adrenal Androgens

- Small contribution to androgen production in males
- ~50% androgens for females
- Clinical relevance: **congenital adrenal hyperplasia**
  - Over/underproduction → abnormal sexual development
- Production stimulated by ACTH (like cortisol)

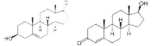

Dehydroepiandrosterone (DHEA)   Testosterone   Androstenedione

Cortisol

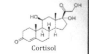

Cortisol

- Major glucocorticoid
- Synthesized by adrenal cortex
- Binds to intracellular receptors (cytosol)
  - **Glucocorticoid receptor (GR)**
- Translocates to nucleus
- Activates/suppresses gene transcription

Pituitary-Adrenal Axis

- Controls **cortisol secretion**
- Hypothalamus: CRH
  - Corticotropin releasing hormone
  - Paraventricular nucleus (PVN)
- Anterior pituitary: ACTH
  - Adrenocorticotropic hormone
  - Acts on adrenal gland
  - cAMP/PKA 2nd messenger
- Adrenal: Cortisol

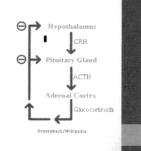

Drosenbach/Wikipedia

Circadian Rhythms

- Serum cortisol **highest early morning** (about 6 AM)
  - 10 to 20 mcg/dL
- Lowest one hour after sleep onset
  - Less than 5 mcg/dL
- Testing rarely done with single blood test

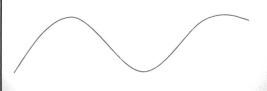

Cortisol Binding Globulin

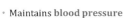

Cortisol

- Cortisol poorly soluble in plasma
- Most (>90%) serum cortisol bound to CBG
- Levels ↑ estrogen

Cortisol
Hormone Effects

- Maintains **blood pressure**
  - Effects on vascular smooth muscle
  - Increases vascular sensitivity (α1) to norepi/epi
  - ↓NO mediated vasodilation
- ↑ cortisol: hypertension (Cushing's disease)
- ↓ cortisol: hypotension (adrenal insufficiency)

Cortisol

Cortisol
Hormone Effects

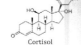
Cortisol

- Suppresses **immune system**
- Sequester lymphocytes in spleen/nodes
  - **Reduce T and B cell levels in plasma**
- Block neutrophil migration
  - ↑ **peripheral neutrophil count**
- Mast cells: blocks histamine release
- ↓ eosinophil counts
- Basis for steroids as immunosuppressive drug therapy

Cortisol

Cortisol

- Inactivate **NF-KB**
  - Key inflammatory transcription factor
  - Mediates response to TNF-α
  - Controls synthesis inflammatory mediators
  - COX-2, PLA2, Lipoxygenase

Corticosteroid Drugs

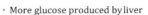

Cortisol

Dexamethasone

Prednisone   Methylprednisolone   Cortisone

Triamcinolone   Betamethasone   Hydrocortiosne

Cortisol
Effects

Cortisol

- More glucose produced by liver
  - ↑ synthesis of glucose 6-phosphatase, PEPCK
  - ↑ **gluconeogenesis**
- Less glucose taken up peripherally (muscle, fat)
- Net results: ↑ **serum glucose**
- More glycogen storage in liver
  - ↑ synthesis of glycogen synthase

Cortisol
Effects

Cortisol

- Activation of lipolysis in adipocytes
  - ↑ free fatty acids
  - ↑ **total cholesterol, ↑ triglycerides**
- Stimulate adipocyte growth
- Key effect: **fat deposition**

Cortisol
Effects

Cortisol

- Enhanced effects of glucagon, epinephrine
- Leads to **insulin resistance**
- Long term steroid use: **diabetes**

Cortisol
Effects

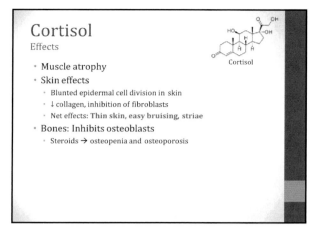

Cortisol

- Muscle atrophy
- Skin effects
  - Blunted epidermal cell division in skin
  - ↓ collagen, inhibition of fibroblasts
  - Net effects: **Thin skin, easy bruising, striae**
- Bones: Inhibits osteoblasts
  - Steroids → osteopenia and osteoporosis

Zones of the Adrenal Glands

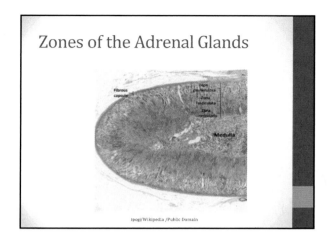

Jpogi/Wikipedia /Public Domain

Zones of the Adrenal Glands

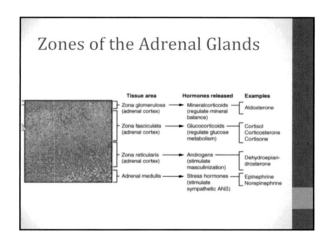

Tissue area	Hormones released	Examples
Zona glomerulosa (adrenal cortex)	Mineralcorticoids (regulate mineral balance)	Aldosterone
Zona fasciculata (adrenal cortex)	Glucocorticoids (regulate glucose metabolism)	Cortisol Corticosterone Cortisone
Zona reticularis (adrenal cortex)	Androgens (stimulate masculinization)	Dehydroepian-drosterone
Adrenal medulla	Stress hormones (stimulate sympathetic ANS)	Epinephrine Norepinephrine

Zona Glomerulosa

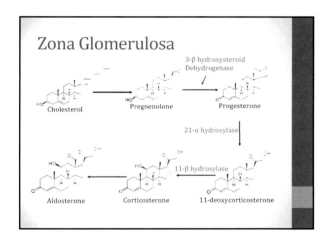

Zona Glomerulosa

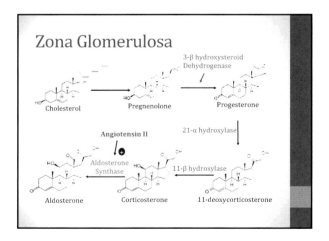

Zona Glomerulosa

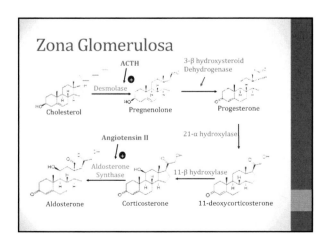

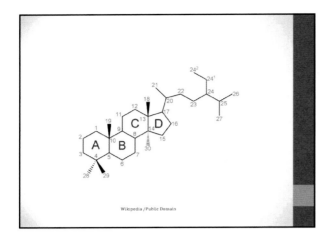

Wikipedia /Public Domain

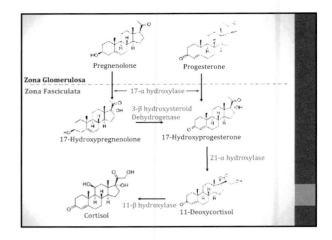

Zona Glomerulosa
Zona Fasciculata

Pregnenolone — Progesterone
17-α hydroxylase
17-Hydroxypregnenolone — 17-Hydroxyprogesterone
3-β hydroxysteroid Dehydrogenase
21-α hydroxylase
11-β hydroxylase
Cortisol — 11-Deoxycortisol

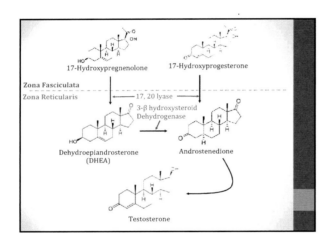

Zona Fasciculata
Zona Reticularis

17-Hydroxypregnenolone — 17-Hydroxyprogesterone
17, 20 lyase
3-β hydroxysteroid Dehydrogenase
Dehydroepiandrosterone (DHEA) — Androstenedione
Testosterone

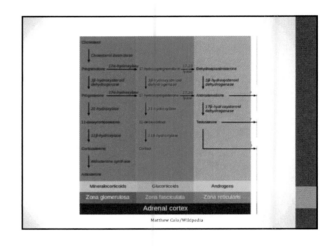

Matthew Colo/Wikipedia

Ketoconazole

- Antifungal
- Blocks ergosterol synthesis in fungi
- Potent inhibitor of 17,20 lyase
  - ↓ androstenedione/testosterone
  - Key side effect: **gynecomastia**
- Also inhibits 17-alpha hydroxylase, desmolase
  - **Blocks cortisol synthesis**
  - Can be used to treat Cushing's syndrome

24

Congenital Adrenal Hyperplasia

Jason Ryan, MD, MPH

CAH
Congenital Adrenal Hyperplasia

- Enzyme deficiency syndrome
- Loss of one of the four enzymes for cortisol synthesis
  - 21-α hydroxylase
  - 11-β hydroxylase
  - 17-α hydroxylase
  - 3-β hydroxysteroid dehydrogenase

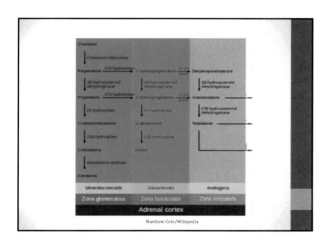

Matthew Colo/Wikipedia

CAH
Congenital Adrenal Hyperplasia

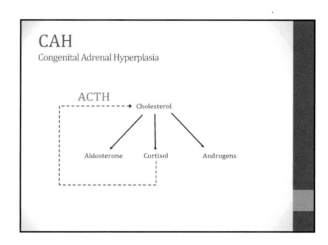

CAH
Congenital Adrenal Hyperplasia

- All result in low cortisol
- Stimulates ACTH release
- Can cause ↑ production of other hormones
  - Mineralocorticoids
  - Androgens

↓ Cortisol ⟶ ↑ACTH ⟶ Adrenal Hyperplasia ⟶ ↑ Non-cortisol hormone synthesis

---

Low Cortisol
Signs/Symptoms

- Hypoglycemia
- Nausea/vomiting

Aldosterone
Signs/Symptoms

- **Deficiency**
  - Na loss → water loss
  - Hypovolemia → shock
  - Hyperkalemia
  - ↑ renin
- **Excess**
  - Na retention
  - Hypertension
  - Hypokalemia
  - ↓ renin

Androgens
Signs/Symptoms

- Depend on chromosomal sex of child (XX/XY)
- Excess androgens
  - Female (XX): **Ambiguous genitalia**
  - Male (XY): Precocious (early) puberty
- Androgen deficiency
  - Female (XX): Normal genitalia
  - Male (XY): Female or ambiguous genitalia

Ambiguous Genitalia

- Females (XX) with excess androgen exposure
- Males (XY) with deficient androgen exposure

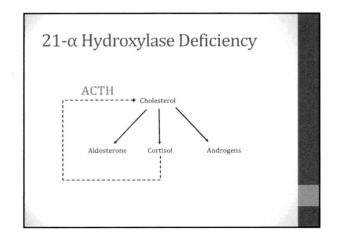

Diabetic fetopathy associated with bilateral adrenal hyperplasia and ambiguous genitalia: a case report.
Journal of Medical Case Reports. 2008: **2** : 251. doi:10.1186/1752-1947-2-251

ACTH Effects

- High ACTH can case **skin hyperpigmentation**
- Melanocyte stimulating hormone (MSH)
  - Common precursor protein in pituitary with ACTH
- ↑ melanin synthesis

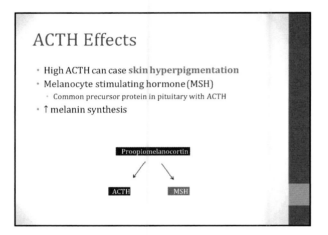

21-α Hydroxylase Deficiency

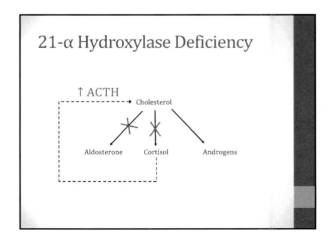

21-α Hydroxylase Deficiency

21-α Hydroxylase Deficiency

- Classic cause of CAH (90% of CAH)
- Low cortisol symptoms
- Low mineralocorticoid symptoms
- Excess androgen symptoms
  - Girls (XX): **ambiguous genitalia**
  - Boys (XY): precocious puberty (early onset)
- Variable symptoms based on enzyme levels
  - Classic form: 0 to 2% normal enzyme activity
  - Non-classic forms: 20-50% normal enzyme activity

21-α Hydroxylase Deficiency

Type	Clinical Features
Classic, Salt-losing	Nausea/Vomiting Volume depletion Hyperkalemia 7 to 14 days
Milder Forms	Females: Ambiguous genitalia Males: Precocious puberty

11-β Hydroxylase Deficiency

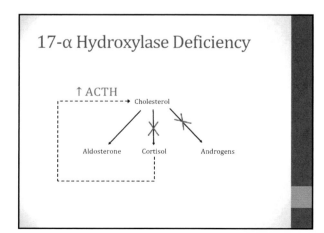

↑ ACTH

Cholesterol

11-deoxycorticosterone

Aldosterone   Cortisol   Androgens

11-β Hydroxylase Deficiency

- Similar to 21-α hydroxylase deficiency
  - Low cortisol symptoms
  - Girls: ambiguous genitalia
  - Boys: precocious puberty
- One exception: ↑ **mineralocorticoid activity**
  - ↑ 11-deoxycorticosterone (weak mineralocorticoid)
- **Hypertension**
- **Hypokalemia**

17-α Hydroxylase Deficiency

↑ ACTH

Cholesterol

Aldosterone   Cortisol   Androgens

17-α Hydroxylase Deficiency

- Cytochrome P450c17 enzyme (CYP17A1)
- Found in adrenal glands and gonads
- Catalyzes two reactions
  - 17-hydroxylase
  - 17,20-lyase

17-α Hydroxylase Deficiency

- Low cortisol
- Excess mineralocorticoids: HTN, ↓K⁺
- Low androgens
  - CYP17A1 : adrenal gland and gonads

17-α Hydroxylase Deficiency

- Males (XY):
  - Female or ambiguous external genitalia
  - Absent uterus/fallopian tubes (Sertoli cells → MIH)
  - Undescended testes

17-α Hydroxylase Deficiency

- Females (XX):
  - Normal at birth
  - Primary amenorrhea at puberty
  - Theca cells lack of androgens → ↓ estradiol
- Often **diagnosed at puberty**
  - XX female fails to develop
  - XY phenotypic female or male fails to develop
  - Hypertension, low K⁺ identified

3-β Hydroxysteroid Dehydrogenase Deficiency

↑ ACTH → Cholesterol

Aldosterone   Cortisol   Androgens

Disorders of Sex Development

Ambiguous Genitalia

46, XX   46, XY

Excess Androgens   **Lack of androgens**
Often CAH   Synthesis/Effect
                      Rarely due to CAH

CAH Screening

- Some states screen with newborn blood testing
- Measure level of **17-Hydroxyprogesterone**
  - Elevated level in 21-α hydroxylase deficiency (most common)

CAH Treatment

- Many forms treated with **glucocorticoids**
- Replenishes cortisol
- Lowers ACTH
- Stops overproduction of other hormones
- Can also use **mineralocorticoids** (fludrocortisone)

Adrenal Disorders

Jason Ryan, MD, MPH

Adrenal Disorders

- Excess cortisol
- Insufficient cortisol
- Excess mineralocorticoids
- Tumors

Cushing's Syndrome

- Syndrome of clinical features due to **excess cortisol**
- Most common cause: **corticosteroid medication**
  - Often prescribed for inflammatory conditions
  - i.e. daily prednisone for lupus
- Cushing's **disease**: Pituitary ACTH-secreting tumor
  - One cause of Cushing's syndrome

Cushing's Syndrome
Excess Cortisol Effects

- Hypertension
- Hyperglycemia
- Diabetes (insulin resistance)
- Immune suppression
  - Risk of infections, especially opportunistic

Cushing's Syndrome
Excess Cortisol Effects

- Cortisol alters GnRH release → ↓ FSH,LH
- Menstrual irregularities in women
  - Abnormal cycles (80%)
  - Oligomenorrhea (~30%)
  - Amenorrhea (~30%)
- Hirsutism of face in women
- Males: Erectile dysfunction

Cushing's Syndrome
Excess Cortisol Effects

- Stimulation of adipocytes → growth
- Progressive central obesity
- Face, neck, trunk, abdomen
- "Moon face"
- "Buffalo hump"
  - Fat mound at base of back of neck

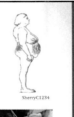

SherryC1234

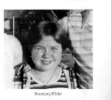

Homini/Flikr

Skin Changes

- Thinning of skin
- Easy bruising
- Striae: Stretch marks
  - Purple lines on skin
  - Fragile skin stretches over trunk, breasts, abdomen
  - Thin skin cannot hide venous blood in dermis
  - Commonly occur on sides and lower abdomen

Cushing's Syndrome
Causes

- ACTH-independent (↓ACTH)
  - **Glucocorticoid therapy**
  - Adrenal adenoma
- ACTH-dependent (↑ACTH)
  - Cushing's disease (pituitary ACTH secreting tumor)
  - Ectopic ACTH (small cell lung cancer)
  - ↑ACTH → **adrenal hyperplasia** → ↑cortisol

Cushing's Syndrome
Causes

- Special note: **skin hyperpigmentation**
  - Can occur in ACTH-dependent Cushing's syndrome
  - Caused by ↑ ACTH not cortisol
  - ↑ ACTH → ↑ MSH

Wikipedia/Public Domain

Cushing's Syndrome
Diagnosis

- Measuring plasma cortisol difficult
- Circadian rhythm → high levels in AM
- Most cortisol bound to CBG
- CBG levels can affect serum measurement

Cushing's Syndrome
Diagnosis

- 24-hour urine free cortisol
  - Integrates cortisol level over time
- Salivary cortisol
  - No cortisol binding globulin in saliva
  - Free cortisol level measured at night (should be low)

Cushing's Syndrome
Diagnosis

- **Low dose dexamethasone suppression test**
  - 1mg dexamethasone ("low dose") administered at bedtime
  - Suppresses normal pituitary ACTH release
  - Morning blood test
  - Cortisol level should be low (suppressed)
  - Cortisol **remains high in Cushing's syndrome**
  - Adenomas, tumors do not suppress cortisol production

Cushing's Syndrome
Diagnosis

- Step 1: Establish Cushing's syndrome
- Step 2: Establish cause
- Key test is serum ACTH level

ACTH-Dependent Causes (High ACTH)	ACTH-Independent Causes (Low ACTH)
Cushing's disease Ectopic ACTH	Steroid therapy Adrenal adenoma

High Dose Dexamethasone

- Low dose testing (1mg)
  - Used to **establish diagnosis** of Cushing's syndrome
- High dose dexamethasone test (3mg)
  - Differentiate causes of high ACTH Cushing's syndrome
  - Will suppress cortisol in pituitary adenomas ($\uparrow$ set point)
  - Will not suppress cortisol from ACTH tumors

AM Cortisol After Dexamethasone

	Low Dose	High Dose
Normal	$\downarrow$	$\downarrow$
Pituitary Adenoma	--	$\downarrow$
ACTH Tumor	--	--

Cushing's Syndrome
Treatment

- **Surgery**
  - Removal of adenoma (adrenal gland, pituitary)
  - Removal of lung tumor
- Ketoconazole

Ketoconazole

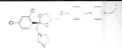

- Antifungal
- Blocks ergosterol synthesis in fungi
- Also **blocks 1st step in cortisol synthesis**
  - Desmolase (side chain cleavage)
- Can be used to treat Cushing's syndrome
- Also potent inhibitor androgen synthesis
  - Key side effect: gynecomastia

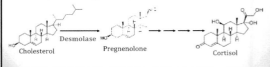

Adrenal Insufficiency

- Insufficient cortisol production
- **Primary** adrenal insufficiency (Addison's disease)
  - Failure of adrenal gland
  - Cortisol and aldosterone will be low
  - ACTH will be high
- **Secondary** adrenal insufficiency
  - Failure of pituitary ACTH release
  - Only cortisol will be low

Adrenal Insufficiency
Symptoms

- Loss of cortisol
  - Weakness, fatigue
  - Weight loss
  - Postural hypotension
  - Nausea, abdominal pain, diarrhea
  - Hypoglycemia
- Loss of aldosterone
  - Potassium retention $\rightarrow$ hyperkalemia
  - H+ retention $\rightarrow$ acidosis
  - Sodium loss in urine $\rightarrow$ hypovolemia

ACTH Effects

- ACTH is high in primary adrenal insufficiency
- This leads to **skin hyperpigmentation**
- Melanocyte stimulating hormone (MSH) shares common precursor protein in pituitary with ACTH
- ↑ melanin synthesis

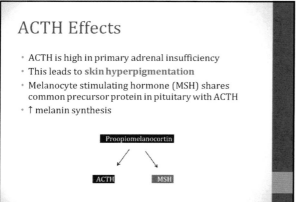

Addison's Hyperpigmentation

- Generalized hyperpigmentation
- Most obvious in sun-exposed areas
  - Face, neck, backs of hands
- Also areas of friction/pressure
  - Elbows, knees, knuckles,
- May occur is palmar creases
- Classic scenario:
  - GI symptoms (nausea, pain)
  - Darkening skin

Wikipedia/Public Domain

Adrenal Crisis

- **Acute** adrenal insufficiency
- Abrupt loss of cortisol and aldosterone
- Main manifestation is **shock**
- Hypoglycemia
- Other symptoms: nausea, vomiting, fatigue, confusion
- Often when acute ↑ adrenal function cannot be met
  - Infection, surgery, trauma in patient with adrenal insufficiency
  - Patients on chronic steroids
  - "Stress dose steroids" for prevention

Addison's Disease
Common Causes

- **Autoimmune adrenalitis**
  - Antibody and cell-mediated disorder
  - Antibodies to 21-hydroxylase commonly seen
  - Atrophy of adrenal gland
  - Loss of cortex
  - Medulla is spared
- **Infections**
  - Tuberculosis
  - Fungal (histoplasmosis, cryptococcus)
  - CMV
- Rare: tumor metastasis especially lung

Metastasis from Lung Cancer

- Adrenals
  - Usually found on imaging without symptoms
- Brain
  - Headache, neuro deficits, seizures
- Bone
  - Pathologic fractures
- Liver
  - Hepatomegaly, jaundice

Waterhouse-Friderichsen Syndrome

- Rare cause of acute adrenal insufficiency
- Caused by acute **hemorrhage** into adrenal glands
- Associated with **meningococcemia**
- Clinical scenario
  - Patient with bacterial meningitis
  - Acute onset of shock

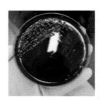

Xishan01/Wikipedia

2° Adrenal Insufficiency

- Most common cause: **glucocorticoid therapy**
- Chronic suppression ACTH release
- Leads to **adrenal atrophy** over time
- Sudden discontinuation → hypoadrenalism

2° Adrenal Insufficiency

- Basis for "weaning" off steroids
  - Slow discontinuation over time
- Basis for "stress dose steroids"
  - Patients on chronic steroids with infection, trauma, surgery
  - Risk of adrenal crisis
  - High dose of glucocorticoids administered

2° Adrenal Insufficiency
Important Points

- No skin findings
  - ACTH is not elevated
- No hyperkalemia
  - Aldosterone not effected

Adrenal Insufficiency
Diagnostic Tests

- 8 AM serum cortisol
  - Levels should be highest at this time
  - Low level indicates disease
- Serum ACTH
  - High ACTH with low cortisol = primary disease
  - Low ACTH with low cortisol = secondary disease

Adrenal Insufficiency
Diagnostic Tests

- ACTH stimulation test ("cosyntropin stim test")
  - Exogenous ACTH administered
  - Cortisol should rise 30-60 minutes later
  - Failure to rise = primary adrenal insufficiency
  - Normal rise = secondary disorder

Primary Aldosteronism
Mineralocorticoid Excess

- **Hypertension**, classically at a young age
- **Hypokalemia**
  - Weakness, muscle cramps
  - Unreliable finding → many cases with normal K+
- **Metabolic alkalosis**

Primary Aldosteronism
Most common causes

- Bilateral idiopathic hyperaldosteronism (~60%)
- Aldosterone-producing adenoma (~30%)
  - Sometimes called Conn's syndrome

Primary Aldosteronism
Diagnosis

- Plasma aldosterone concentration (PAC)
- **Plasma renin activity (PRA)**
  - Plasma incubated
  - Renin cleaves angiotensinogen in plasma
  - Angiotensin I produced → measured by assay
- ↓ PRA and ↑ PAC = Primary aldosteronism
- ↑ PRA and ↑ PAC = Secondary aldosteronism
  - Renal artery stenosis, CHF, low volume

Primary Aldosteronism
Diagnosis

- Abdominal imaging for adrenal nodules/tumors
- **Adrenal vein sampling**
  - Differentiates unilateral vs. bilateral disease
  - Measure PAC and PRA in each vein

Primary Aldosteronism
Treatment

- Surgical adrenalectomy
  - Adenomas
  - Unilateral hyperplasia
- **Spironolactone**
  - Drug of choice
  - Potassium-sparing diuretic
  - Blocks aldosterone effects

Licorice

- Contains glycyrrhetinic acid (a steroid)
  - Weak mineralocorticoid effect
  - Inhibits renal 11-beta-hydroxysteroid dehydrogenase   *Pikaluk/Flikr*
- Large amounts → Hypertension, hypokalemia
- Plasma aldosterone level low

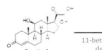

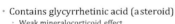

Cortisol   →   11-beta-hydroxysteroid dehydrogenase   →   Cortisone

Pheochromocytoma

- Catecholamine-secreting tumor
  - Secrete epinephrine, norepinephrine, dopamine
- **Chromaffin cells** of adrenal medulla
  - Derivatives of **neural crest**

Pheochromocytoma

- Clinical presentation
  - Classically **episodic** symptoms
  - Hypertension
  - Headaches
  - Palpitations
  - Sweating
  - Pallor (pale skin)

Pheochromocytoma
Diagnosis

- Serum catecholamine levels not routinely used
  - Levels fluctuate
  - Some metabolism intratumoral
- Breakdown products of catecholamines measured
  - Usually via 24 hour urine collection

Pheochromocytoma
Diagnosis

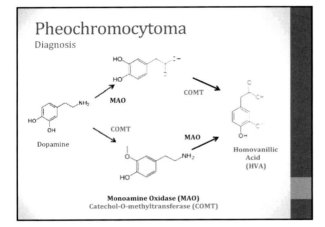

Monoamine Oxidase (MAO)
Catechol-O-methyltransferase (COMT)

Pheochromocytoma
Diagnosis

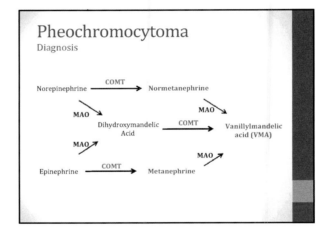

Pheochromocytoma
Diagnosis

- **Metanephrines** often measured for diagnosis
  - Metanephrine and normetanephrine
  - 24 hour urine collection or plasma
- Older test: 24 hour collection of VMA

Pheochromocytoma
Treatment

- Definitive therapy: Surgery
- Pre-operative management:
  - **Phenoxybenzamine** (irreversible α blocker)
  - Non-selective beta blockers (propranolol)

Paraganglioma

- Catecholamine-secreting tumor
- Arise from sympathetic ganglia (extraadrenal)
- Similar clinical presentation to pheochromocytoma

Neuroblastoma

- Tumor of primitive **sympathetic ganglion cells**
  - Also derived from neural crest cells
- Can arise anywhere in sympathetic nervous system
  - Adrenal gland most common (40 percent)
  - Abdominal (25 percent)
  - Thoracic (15 percent)
- Almost always occurs in **children**
  - 3rd most common childhood cancer (leukemia, brain tumors)
  - Most common extracranial tumor

Neuroblastoma

- Symptoms related to tumor mass effect
  - Commonly present as abdominal pain
- Can synthesize catecholamines
  - Rarely cause symptoms like pheochromocytoma
  - **Urinary HVA/VMA levels** used for diagnosis
- Rare feature: Opsoclonus-myoclonus-ataxia (OMA)
  - Rare paraneoplastic syndrome
  - Rapid eye movements, rhythmic jerking, ataxia
  - Half of OMA patients have a neuroblastoma

Neuroblastoma

- Diverse range of disease progression
- Key risk factor: **Age at diagnosis**
  - Infants with disseminated disease often cured
  - Children over 18 months often die despite therapy
  - Younger age = better prognosis
- **N-myc**
  - Proto-oncogene
  - **Amplified/overexpressed** in some tumors
  - Associated with poor prognosis

MIBG
Metaiodobenzylguanidine

- Chemical **analog of norepinephrine**
- Diagnosis of pheochromocytoma & neuroblastoma
- Concentrated in sympathetic tissues
- Labeled with radioactive iodine (I^{131})
- Will **concentrate in tumors** → emit radiation
- Special note: thyroid gland must be protected
  - Simultaneous administration of **potassium iodide**
  - Non-radioactive iodine
  - Will be taken up by thyroid instead

Adrenal Adenomas

- Often discovered on abdominal imaging
  - "Adrenal incidentaloma"
- Concern for malignancy and/or functioning adenoma

Adrenal Adenomas

- May secrete cortisol or aldosterone
- Common functional tests
  - 24 hour urine metanephrines (pheochromocytoma)
  - 24 hour urine free cortisol (Cushing's)
  - Low dose dexamethasone suppression (Cushing's)
  - Serum PRA/aldosterone (aldosteronism)
- Often followed for growth over time (non-functional)
- Large (>5cm) often removed

Endocrine Pancreas

Jason Ryan, MD, MPH

Pancreatic Islets

Islets of Langerhans

- Millions of islets found in pancreatic tissue
- Endocrine portion of pancreas
- Beta cells: Insulin
  - Most abundant cell type
  - Centrally located
- Alpha cells: Glucagon
- Delta cells: Somatostatin
- Alpha/delta cells: Outer islet

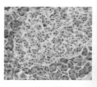

Polarlys/Wikipedia

Insulin

- Protein hormone
- Synthesized by **beta cells**
- Synthesized as preproinsulin
  - Made by ribosomes of rough endoplasmic reticulum
- Preproinsulin cleaved to proinsulin
  - Transported to Golgi apparatus
- Packaged into secretory granules
  - Proinsulin cleaved to insulin and C-peptide in granules

Insulin Structure

- Alpha chain
- Beta chain
- Disulfide bridges
- C-peptide
  - "Connecting" peptide
  - Long half-life
  - Indicator insulin production

C-peptide

α chain

β chain

Zapyon/Wikipedia

Insulin Release

GLUT-2 and Glucokinase
Both in liver/pancreas

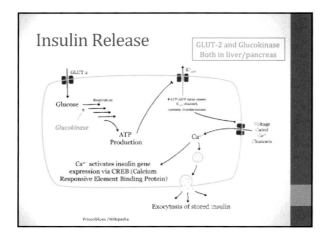

Prisonblues /Wikipedia

Insulin Release

- Produced in response to: **glucose, amino acids**

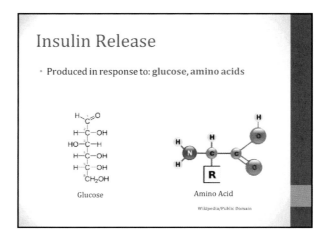

Glucose

Amino Acid

Wikipedia/Public Domain

Insulin Release

- Production **inhibited by epinephrine**
  - Beta-2 receptors: ↑ insulin
  - Alpha-2 receptors: ↓ insulin release
  - Alpha effect is dominant effect in pancreas
  - Fight or flight response → ↑ plasma glucose

Glucokinase

- **Beta cell** enzyme
- 1st step of glycolysis
- Found in liver and pancreas
- Induced by insulin
- Insulin promotes transcription
- High Km (rate varies with glucose)
- High Vm (can convert lots of glucose)

Glucose
ATP
ADP
Glucose-6-phosphate

GLUT-2 Transporter

- **Bidirectional** glucose transporter
- Found in liver, kidney, beta cells
  - Liver, kidney: Gluconeogenesis
  - Beta cells: Glucose in/out based on plasma levels
- Also found in intestine, other tissues

Insulin Release
Key Points

- Glucose into beta cells via GLUT-2
- Glucose → G-6P via glucokinase
- ATP produced → Closure of K⁺ channels
- Depolarization
- Voltage-gated calcium channels open
- Calcium → insulin release from vesicles

Insulin Receptor

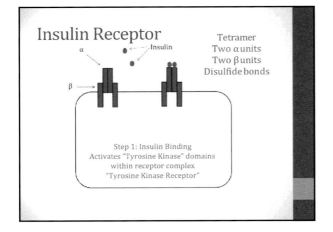

Tetramer
Two α units
Two β units
Disulfide bonds

Step 1: Insulin Binding
Activates "Tyrosine Kinase" domains
within receptor complex
"Tyrosine Kinase Receptor"

Insulin Receptor

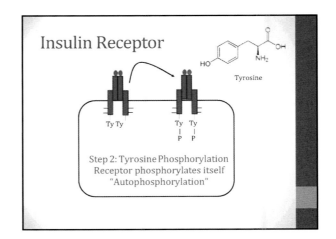

Step 2: Tyrosine Phosphorylation
Receptor phosphorylates itself
"Autophosphorylation"

Insulin Receptor

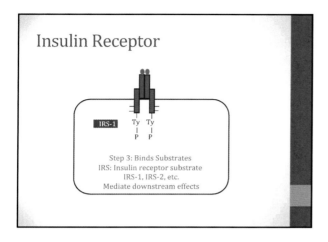

Step 3: Binds Substrates
IRS: Insulin receptor substrate
IRS-1, IRS-2, etc.
Mediate downstream effects

Insulin Receptor

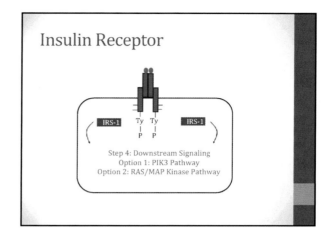

Step 4: Downstream Signaling
Option 1: PIK3 Pathway
Option 2: RAS/MAP Kinase Pathway

PIK3 Pathway
Phosphatidylinositol 3–kinase Pathway

- Intracellular lipid kinases
- Phosphorylate 3'-hydroxyl group of phospholipids
  - Forms PIP_3 from PIP_2

Phosphatidylinositol

PIK3 Pathway
Phosphatidylinositol 3–kinase Pathway

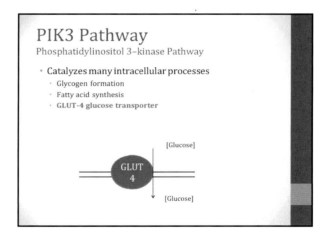

- Catalyzes many intracellular processes
  - Glycogen formation
  - Fatty acid synthesis
  - **GLUT-4 glucose transporter**

[Glucose]

GLUT 4

[Glucose]

GLUT-4 Transporter

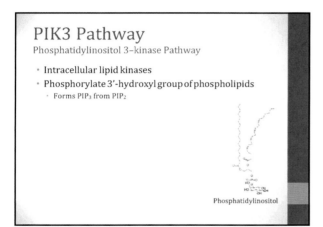

- Stored in vesicles in cells, especially muscle
- Insulin → PIK3 pathway → GLUT-4 Activation
- Major mechanism for increased glucose uptake
- Important muscle/fat
- Insulin exposure → GLUT-4 on surface

[Glucose]

GLUT 4

[Glucose]

RAS/MAP Kinase Pathway

- Insulin receptor can activate RAS
  - G protein
- RAS can activate many growth pathways
  - Raf
  - MEK (mitogen-activated extracellular kinase)
  - MAP (mitogen-activated protein)
- Modify **cell growth** and **gene expression**

Insulin Receptor
Key Points

- Tetramer of α/β subunits with disulfide bridges
  - α: extracellular
  - β: transmembrane
- Insulin binding → **tyrosine kinase** activity
- Autophosphorylation of tyrosine residues
- PIK3 Pathway → **GLUT-4 glucose transporter**
- RAS/MAP Kinase Pathway: growth/gene transcription

Insulin Dependent Organs

- Muscle and fat
  - Use GLUT-4 for glucose uptake
  - Depend on insulin (no insulin = no GLUT-4)

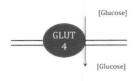

Insulin Independent Organs

- Brain and RBCs
  - Use **GLUT-1** for glucose uptake
  - Not dependent on insulin
  - Takes up glucose when available
  - RBCs: No mitochondria (depend on glycolysis)
  - Brain: No fatty acid metabolism (glucose/ketones)
- Liver, kidney, intestines
  - Also insulin independent (GLUT-2)
- Other organs: nerves, lens

Insulin Effects

- Glucose uptake (skeletal muscle, adipose tissue)
- **Glycogen synthesis**
  - Activates glycogen synthase
  - Inhibits glycogen phosphorylase
- **Inhibits gluconeogenesis**
  - ↑ Fructose-2,6-bisphosphate levels
  - Inhibit Fructose 1,6 bisphosphatase 1

Insulin Effects

- **Fatty acid synthesis**
  - Activates acetyl-CoA carboxylase
  - Inhibits hormone sensitive lipase
- **Protein synthesis**
  - Stimulates entry of amino acids into cells → protein synthesis
  - Important for muscle growth
- Key side effect insulin therapy: weight gain

Hormone Sensitive Lipase

- Removes fatty acids from TAG in adipocytes
- Inhibited by **insulin**
- Activated by **glucagon** and **epinephrine**

Triacylglycerol

Fatty Acid

Hormone Sensitive Lipase

Glycerol → Liver

Insulin Effects

- Na+ retention
  - Increases Na+ resorption in the nephron
- **Lowers potassium**
  - Enhanced activity of Na-K-ATPase pump in skeletal muscle
  - Insulin plus glucose used in treatment of **hyperkalemia**
- Inhibits glucagon release

Glucagon

- Protein hormone
- Single polypeptide chain
- Synthesized by **alpha cells**
- Opposes actions of insulin
- Main stimulus release: low plasma glucose

Glucagon

- Increases liver (not muscle) **glycogen breakdown**
  - Raises blood glucose level
- Increases **gluconeogenesis**

Glucagon

- Increases **amino acid uptake in liver**
  - More carbon skeletons for glucose via gluconeogenesis
  - Plasma amino acid levels fall
- Activates lipolysis via **hormone sensitive lipase**

Glucagon Receptor

- **G-protein receptor**
- Activates adenylyl cyclase
- Increases **cAMP**
- Activates protein kinase A (PKA)

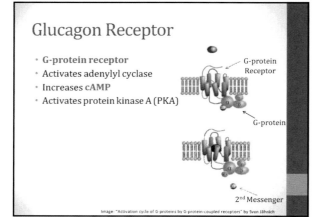

G-protein Receptor

G-protein

2nd Messenger

Image: "Activation cycle of G-proteins by G-protein-coupled receptors" by Sven Jähnich

Glucagon Receptor

- **Glucagon receptors mostly in liver**
  - Many activated processes occur in liver
  - Breakdown of glycogen to raise plasma glucose
  - Gluconeogenesis
- Most other tissues have lower density than liver
- Not found in skeletal muscle

Watanabe M, et al. Histologic distribution of insulin and glucagon receptors. Brazilian Journal of Medical and Biological Research (1998) 31: 243-256

Hypoglycemia

- Unconscious patient with hypoglycemia
- Treatment:
  - #1: IV dextrose
  - #2: Intramuscular glucagon
- Useful when IV access cannot be established
- Raises plasma glucose level

Beta Blocker Overdose

- Causes bradycardia and hypotension
- Drug of choice: **Glucagon**
  - Activates adenylyl cyclase
  - Different site from beta-adrenergic agents
  - Raises cAMP → ↑ myocyte calcium
  - Same mechanism as beta stimulation (via Gs proteins)

Insulinoma

- Rare, pancreatic islet-cell tumor
- Occurs in adults (median age ~50 years)
- Key feature: **fasting hypoglycemia**
  - Insulin levels remain elevated when fasting
- "Neuroglycopenic symptoms"
  - Confusion, odd behavior
- Sympathetic activation from low glucose
  - Palpitations, diaphoresis, tremor

Insulinoma

- Diagnosis: fasting insulin level
- Also elevated
  - C-peptide
  - Proinsulin
- Need to exclude exogenous insulin administration

Fasting Hypoglycemia

- Differential diagnosis
  - Exogenous insulin
  - Oral hypoglycemics (sulfonylureas → ↑ insulin)
  - Insulinoma

	Exogenous Insulin	Insulinoma	Oral Hypoglycemics
Insulin	+	+	+
C-peptide	--	+	+
Hypoglycemic Agent Screen	--	--	+

Glucagonoma

- Rare pancreatic tumors
- Excess glucagon secretion
- Leads to **glucose intolerance**
  - Elevated fasting glucose levels
  - Rare to develop DKA (insulin function intact)

Glucagonoma

- **Weight loss**
  - Liver gluconeogenesis
  - Consumption of proteins/amino acids

Glucagonoma

- **Necrolytic migratory erythema**
  - Red, blistering rash
  - Itchy, painful
  - Fluctuates in severity
  - **Genitals, buttocks, groin**
- Key clinical scenario: **new diabetes and rash**

Glucagonoma

- Diagnosis: ↑ plasma glucagon level
- Treatment: **somatostatin analogs** (octreotide)
  - Inhibit glucagon secretion
  - Improves symptoms

MEN Syndromes

- Multiple endocrine neoplasia
- Rare inherited disorders
- Numerous endocrine tumors
- **MEN Type 1**: Insulinomas/glucagonomas
  - 3 P's: Pituitary, Parathyroid, and Pancreas
  - Mutations of MEN1 tumor suppressor gene

Diabetes

Jason Ryan, MD, MPH

Diabetes

- Chronic disorder of elevated blood glucose levels
- Caused by:
  - Insufficient insulin
  - Insufficient response to insulin ("insulin resistance")
  - Both

Diabetes Symptoms

- Often asymptomatic
  - "Silent killer"
  - Often no symptoms until complications develop
  - Basis for screening
- Classic hyperglycemia symptoms
  - Polyuria (osmotic diuresis from glucose)
  - Polydipsia (thirst to replace lost fluids)

Terminology

- Diabetes Mellitus
  - Mellitus = sweet
  - Common disorder of blood glucose
- Diabetes insipidus
  - Insipid = lacking flavor
  - Rare disorder of low ADH activity
- Both can cause polyuria, polydipsia
- Completely different mechanisms

Diabetes Diagnosis

- Symptoms
  - Symptoms plus glucose >200mg/dl = diabetes
- Asymptomatic
  - Fasting blood glucose level (no food for 8 hours)

State	Fasting plasma glucose
Normal	<100mgl/dl
Pre-diabetes	100 to 125mg/dl
Diabetes	>=126mg/dl

Hemoglobin A1C

- Small fraction of hemoglobin is "glycated"
  - Glucose combines with alpha/beta chains
- Subfraction HbA1c used in diabetes
  - Non-enzymatic glycation of beta-chains
  - Occurs at amino-terminal valines

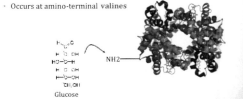

Glucose

NH2

Hemoglobin A1C

- Reflects average glucose over past 3 months
  - Normal < 5.7%
  - Pre-diabetes: 5.7 to 6.4%
  - Diabetes: >=6.5%
- Sometimes used for diagnosis
- Important for monitoring therapy
  - Higher value = worse control of blood sugar

Glucose Tolerance Test

- Oral glucose load administered
- Plasma glucose measured 1-3 hours later
- High glucose indicates diabetes
- Often used to screen for **gestational diabetes**
  - Some insulin resistance normal in pregnancy
  - Need to study response to glucose load for diagnosis

Type 1 Diabetes

- Autoimmune disorder
- **Type IV hypersensitivity** reaction
- T-cell mediated destruction of beta cells
  - Inflammation of islets
  - **Lymphocytes** on biopsy ("Insulitis")
  - Decreased number of beta cells
  - **Loss of insulin**
- Associated with HLA-DR3 and HLA-DR4
- Autoantibodies may be present
  - Islet-cell antibodies
  - Insulin antibodies

Type 1 Diabetes

Wikipedia/Public Domain

- Mostly a **childhood disorder**
  - Bimodal distribution
  - Peak at 4-6 years
  - 2nd peak 10 to 14 years of age
- Often presents with symptomatic hyperglycemia
  - Polyuria
  - Polydipsia
  - Glucose in urine
- Treatment: **Insulin**

Diabetic Ketoacidosis
DKA

- Life-threatening complication of diabetes
- More common type 1
- Common **initial presentation** type 1
- Often precipitated by infection/trauma
- Can occur when type 1 diabetic **skips insulin therapy**

Diabetic Ketoacidosis
DKA

Diabetic Ketoacidosis
Clinical Presentation

- Abdominal pain/nausea/vomiting
- Dehydration
- Hyperglycemia
- Hyperkalemia
- Elevated plasma/urine ketones
- Glucose in urine
- Anion gap metabolic acidosis
  - Kussmaul breathing: deep, labored breathing
  - Hyperventilation to blow off CO2 and raise pH
- Fruity smell on breath

Diabetic Ketoacidosis
DKA

- Low insulin/high epinephrine
- High fatty acid utilization
- Oxaloacetate depleted → TCA cycle stalls
- ↑ acetyl-CoA
- Ketone production

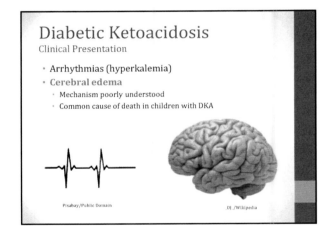

Phosphate

- Risk of **hypophosphatemia**
  - Acidosis → shifts phosphate to extracellular fluid
  - Phosphaturia caused by osmotic diuresis
- Loss of ATP
  - Muscle weakness (respiratory failure)
  - Heart failure (↓ contractility)

6 C	7 N	8 O
14 Si	15 P	16 S
32 Ge	33 As	34 Se

Diabetic Ketoacidosis
Clinical Presentation

- Arrhythmias (hyperkalemia)
- **Cerebral edema**
  - Mechanism poorly understood
  - Common cause of death in children with DKA

Pixabay/Public Domain

DJ /Wikipedia

Mucormycosis

- **Fungal infection**
- Caused by **Rhizopus** sp. and **Mucor** sp.
- Classically starts in sinuses
- Spreads to adjacent structures
- Thrives in high glucose, ketoacidosis conditions
- Classic complication of DKA
  - Patient with DKA
  - Fever, headache, eye pain

Image courtesy of Yale Rose/Flickr

Diabetic Ketoacidosis
Treatment

- **Insulin**
  - Lowers blood glucose levels
  - Shifts potassium into cells
- **IV fluids**
  - Treats dehydration

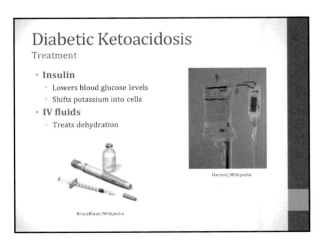

Harmid/Wikipedia

BruceBlaus/Wikipedia

Diabetic Ketoacidosis
Treatment

- Careful monitoring potassium
  - **Total body potassium is low** despite hyperkalemia
  - Insulin shifts into cells → can lead to hypokalemia
  - Usually need to administer potassium
- Careful monitoring glucose
  - Continue insulin until acidosis resolves
  - Often add glucose while insulin infusion continues

Type 2 Diabetes

- **Insulin resistance**
  - Muscle, adipose tissue, liver
- Reduced response to insulin → hyperglycemia
- Pancreas responds with ↑ insulin
- Eventually pancreas can fail → ↓ insulin

Type 2 Diabetes
Risk Factors

- Most common form of diabetes
- Common in **adults**
  - Prevalence is rising
  - Also becoming more common among children

Type 2 Diabetes
Risk Factors

- Major risk factor: **Obesity**
  - Central or abdominal obesity carries greatest risk
- Intra-abdominal (visceral) fat > subcutaneous fat
  - Visceral fat breakdown less inhibited by insulin
  - More lipolysis → more free fatty acids
  - Decreased glucose transport into cells
- "Apple shape" worse than "pear shape"
  - Apple shape due to increased visceral adipose tissue
  - More subcutaneous adipose tissue in pear shape
- Weight loss improves glucose levels

Type 2 Diabetes
Risk Factors

- Major risk factor: **Obesity**
  - Central or abdominal obesity carries greatest risk
- Intra-abdominal (visceral) fat > subcutaneous fat
  - Visceral fat breakdown less inhibited by insulin
  - More lipolysis → more **free fatty acids**
  - Decreased glucose transport into cells
- "Apple shape" worse than "pear shape"
  - Apple shape due to increased visceral adipose tissue
  - More subcutaneous adipose tissue in pear shape
- Weight loss improves glucose levels

Type 2 Diabetes
Risk Factors

- **Family history**
  - Strong genetic component (more than type I)
  - Any first degree relative with T2DM: ↑ 2-3x risk

Type 2 Diabetes
Insulin Resistance Mechanism

- Reason for insulin resistance not known
- Many data suggest **insulin receptor abnormalities**
- Fatty acids may activate **serine-threonine kinases**
  - Phosphorylate amino acids on beta chain of insulin receptors
  - Inhibiting tyrosine phosphorylation
- ↑ **TNF-α** may be synthesized by adipocytes
  - TNF-α can activate serine-threonine kinases

Serine   Threonine

Type 2 Diabetes
Histology

- Classic finding is **amyloid** in pancreatic islets
- **Amylin** peptide normally made by beta cells
  - Precise function not known
  - Packaged and secreted with insulin
  - Pramlintide: amylin analog used for diabetes treatment
- Accumulates in islets in patients with type 2 diabetes

HHS
Hyperglycemic Hyperosmolar Syndrome

- Life-threatening complication of diabetes
- More common type 2
- High glucose → diuresis
  - Markedly elevated glucose (can be >1000)
- Severe dehydration
- Different from DKA
  - Few or no ketone bodies (insulin present)
  - Usually no acidosis
  - **Very high serum osmolarity → CNS dysfunction**

HHS
Hyperglycemic Hyperosmolar Syndrome

- Polyuria, polydipsia
- Dehydration
- **Mental status changes**
  - Confusion
  - Coma
- Treatment similar to DKA (insulin, IVF)

Acanthosis Nigricans

- Hyperpigmented plaques on skin
- Intertriginous sites (folds)
- Classically neck and axillae
- Associated with **insulin resistance**
  - Often seen obesity, diabetes
- Rarely associated with malignancy
  - Gastric adenocarcinoma most common

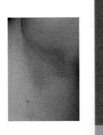

Madhero88/Dermnet.com

Diabetic Complications

- Chronic hyperglycemia → complications
  - Cardiac disease
  - Renal failure
  - Neuropathy
  - Blindness
- **Two key underlying mechanisms**
  - Non-enzymatic glycation
  - Sorbitol accumulation

Non-enzymatic Glycation

- Glucose added to amino groups on proteins
- No enzyme required
- Driven by high glucose levels
- Leads to crosslinked proteins
- "Advanced glycosylation end products" (AGEs)

Atherosclerosis
Diabetic Macroangiopathy

- AGEs trap LDL in large vessels → atherosclerosis
- **Coronary artery disease**
  - Angina, myocardial infarction
- **Stroke/TIA**
- **Peripheral vascular disease**
  - Claudication
  - Arterial ulcers
  - Poor wound healing
  - Gangrene

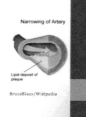

Narrowing of Artery

Lipid deposit of plaque

BruceBlaus/Wikipedia

Diabetic Kidney Disease
Diabetic Microangiopathy

- AGEs → damage to **glomerulus** and **arterioles**
- Leads to **end stage kidney disease** in many diabetics

Diabetic Kidney Disease
Diabetic Microangiopathy

AGEs

Afferent Arteriole

Basement Membrane Thickening

Efferent Arteriole

↓ RBF → Glomerulosclerosis ← Hyperfiltration

Renal Failure

Albuminuria

Renal Arterioles

- Hyaline arteriosclerosis
  - Thickening of arterioles
  - Also seen in HTN
- Can result from AGEs
  - Crosslinking of collagen
- Commonly occurs in **kidneys** of diabetics
  - Can involve afferent **AND efferent** arteriole
  - Afferent arteriole: Ischemia
  - Efferent arteriole: Hyperfiltration
  - Efferent arteriosclerosis rarely seen except in diabetes

Nephron/Wikipedia

Proteinuria in Diabetics

- Annual screening for albumin in urine
- Evidence of protein is indication for **ACE-inhibitor**
- ACEi shown to reduce progression to ESRD
  - Potential mechanism is dilation of efferent arteriole
  - Reduction in hyperfiltration

Glomerular Basement Membranes

- AGEs → diffuse **basement membrane thickening**
- Visible on electron microscopy
- Can lead to mesangial proliferation in glomeruli
- End result is glomerulosclerosis

Glomerulosclerosis

- Diffuse glomerulosclerosis
  - Deposits of proteins (collagen IV)
  - Diffusely on basement membranes of glomeruli capillary loops
  - Mesangial cell proliferation
  - Also occurs with aging and hypertension
  - If severe → **nephrotic syndrome**
- **Nodular** glomerulosclerosis
  - Nodules form in periphery of glomerulus in mesangium
  - Rarely occurs except in diabetes
- Can lead to fibrosis/scarring of entire kidney

Kimmelstiel-Wilson Nodules

- Hallmark of nodular sclerosis of diabetes
- Pathognomonic of diabetic kidney disease

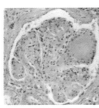

bilalbanday

Sorbitol Accumulation
Polyol Pathway

$$Glucose \xrightarrow[\substack{Aldose \\ Reductase}]{\substack{NADPH \quad NADP+}} Sorbitol \xrightarrow[\substack{Sorbitol \\ Dehydrogenase}]{\substack{NAD+ \quad NADH}} Fructose$$

Polyol Pathway

- Little activity at physiologic glucose levels
- Chronic hyperglycemia can lead to ↑sorbitol
- Sorbitol is osmotic agent
- Draws in fluid → **osmotic damage**
- Likely involved in many diabetic complications
  - Cataracts
  - Neuropathy

Cataracts

- Sorbitol accumulates in **lens**
- ↑ osmolarity
- Fluid into lens
- Opacification over time

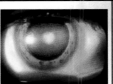

Rakesh Ahuja, MD/Wikipedia

Neuropathy

- **Sorbitol can accumulate in Schwann cells**
  - Myelinating cells of peripheral nerves
  - Osmotic damage → neuropathy

Neuropathy

- Classically causes "stocking-glove" sensory loss
  - Longest axons affected most
  - Often feet/legs
  - Worse distally; better proximally
- Loss of **vibration sense, proprioception**
- Impairment of pain, light touch, temperature
- **Autonomic neuropathy**
  - Postural hypotension
  - Delayed gastric emptying

Diabetic Foot Disease

- Neuropathy + ischemia can lead to:
  - Ulcers
  - Infection
  - **Amputation**
- Made worse by poor wound healing from PVD
- Prevention: **Regular foot exams**
- Ulcer treatment:
  - Wound management
  - Sometimes antibiotics
  - Hyperbaric oxygen chamber

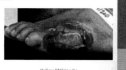

DrGnu/Wikipedia

Diabetic Retinopathy

- Can cause blindness among diabetics
- Multiple factors likely involved:
  - Capillary basement membrane thickening (AGEs)
  - Hyaline arteriosclerosis
- **Pericyte degeneration**
  - Cells that wrap capillaries
  - Evidence of sorbitol accumulation
  - **Microaneurysms**
  - Rupture → **hemorrhage**
- Annual screening for prevention

Diabetic Retinopathy
Findings

- Microaneurysms, Hemorrhages
  - Loss of pericytes
- Exudates
  - Leakage proteins, lipids
- Cotton-wool spots
  - Nerve infarctions
  - Occlusion of precapillary arterioles
- Vessel proliferation ("proliferative retinopathy")
  - Retinal ischemia → new vessel growth
  - "Neovascularization"

"Blausen gallery 2014"
Wikiversity Journal of Medicine.

Diabetes Complications

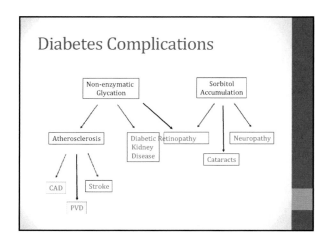

Type 1 versus Type 2

	Type 1	Type 2
Pathophysiology	Loss of insulin	Insulin Resistance
Insulin	Low	High then low
Biopsy	Insulitis	Amyloid
Age	Children	Adults
Genetic Predisposition	Weaker	Stronger
Complications	DKA	HHS

Insulin

Jason Ryan, MD, MPH

Type 1 and Type 2

- Type 1 diabetes treated mainly with insulin
- Type 2 diabetes: **oral or SQ drugs +/-insulin**
  - Initial stages: Oral and/or SQ drugs
  - Advanced disease: Insulin

Insulin

- Many different types available for diabetes therapy
- All vary by **time to peak** and **duration of action**
- Also vary by peak effect

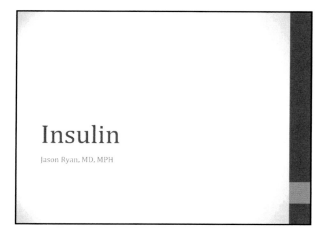

| Rapid Acting Insulin | Regular Insulin | NPH Insulin | Detemir | Glargine |

Fast Peak / Short Duration ———→ Slow Peak / Long Duration

Insulin Hexamers

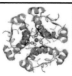

- Insulin forms **hexamers** in the body
  - Six insulin molecules linked
  - Stable structure

  Isaac Yonemoto /Wikipedia

- Insulin usually administered **subcutaneously**
- Activity related to speed of absorption
- Insulin hexamers → slower onset of action
- Insulin monomers → faster onset of action

Rapid Acting Insulin
Lispro, Aspart, and Glulisine

- Modified human insulin
- Contain insulin with modified amino acids
- **Reduced hexamer/polymer formation**
- Rapid absorption, faster action, shorter duration
  - Onset: 15 minutes
  - Peak: 1 hour
  - Duration: 2 to 4 hours
- Often used **pre-meal**

Insulin

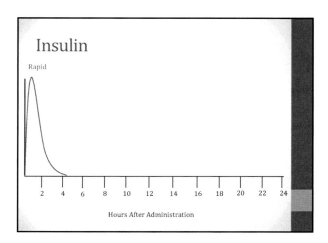

Rapid

Hours After Administration

Regular Insulin

- Synthetic analog of **human insulin**
- Made by recombinant DNA techniques
- Onset: 30 minutes
- Peak: 2 to 3 hours
- Duration: 3 to 6 hours

Insulin

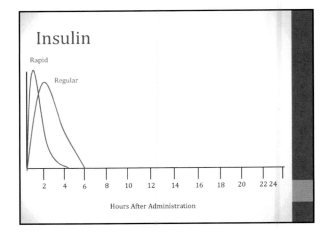

Regular Insulin

- Commonly used in hospitalized patients
  - Blood sugar elevations common with infection/surgery
  - Sliding scale dose given based on finger stick blood sugar
  - "Regular insulin sliding scale"
- Only type of insulin that is given IV
- IV regular insulin used in **DKA/HHS**
- Used to treat **hyperkalemia**
  - Given IV with glucose to prevent hypoglycemia

NPH Insulin
Neutral Protamine Hagedorn

- Regular insulin combined with **neutral protamine**
- Slows absorption
- Peak: 4-8 hours
- Duration: 12-16 hours

Insulin

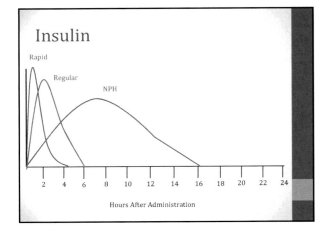

Glargine

- Insulin with modified amino acid structure
- Soluble in acidic solution for dosing
- **Precipitates at body pH** after SQ injection
- Insulin molecules slowly dissolve from crystals
- Low, continuous level of insulin
  - Onset: 1–1.5 hours
  - Duration: 11–24 hours
- Often given **once daily**

Insulin

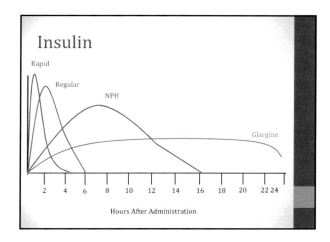

Rapid
Regular
NPH
Glargine

Hours After Administration

Detemir

- Insulin with **fatty acid side chain** added
- Slow rate of absorption
  - Aggregation in subcutaneous tissue
  - Also **binds reversibly to albumin**
- Onset: 1–2 hours
- Duration: > 12 hours
- Usually given **once or twice daily**
- May cause less weight gain

Insulin

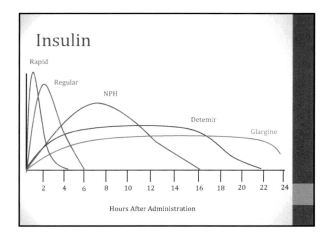

Rapid
Regular
NPH
Detemir
Glargine

Hours After Administration

Insulin

- Rapid-acting
  - Pre-meal
- Regular
  - Sliding scale
  - IV for treatment of DKA, hyperkalemia
- NPH, Glargine, Detemir
  - Often given as background therapy

Insulin Analogs

- Do not contain human insulin molecules
  - Modified insulin structure
  - Rapid acting, Detemir, Glargine
- Regular insulin, NPH
  - Contain human insulin molecules
  - Regular: made by recombinant techniques
  - NPH: Regular added to neutral protamine to slow absorption

Hypoglycemia

- Major side effect of all insulin regimens
  - Tremor, palpitations, sweating, anxiety
  - If severe: seizure, coma
- **Always check blood sugar in unconscious patients**
- Dosages, frequency adjusted to avoid low glucose

Weight Gain

- Occurs in most patients on insulin
- Insulin promotes fatty acid and protein synthesis

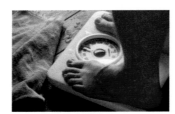

Wikipedia/Public Domain

Treatment of Diabetes

Jason Ryan, MD, MPH

Type 1 and Type 2

- Type 1 diabetes treated mainly with insulin
- Type 2 diabetes: **oral or SQ drugs +/-insulin**
  - Initial stages: Oral and/or SQ drugs
  - Advanced disease: Insulin

Hemoglobin A1C

- Used to monitor therapy
- Too high = ↑ complications
- Too low = Risk of hypoglycemia
- Goal of ≤7.0% often used in many patients

Lifestyle Modifications

- Newly diagnosed type 2 diabetes
- **Weight loss, exercise** improve glucose levels
- First line treatment usually **lifestyle modification**
  - Usually a 3-6 month trial if initial A1c not markedly ↑

Oral/SQ Antidiabetic Agents

- Biguanides (Metformin)
- Sulfonylureas/Meglitinides
- Glitazones
- Glucosidase Inhibitors
- Amylin Analogs
- GLP-1 Analogs
- DPP-4 Inhibitors
- SGLT2 inhibitors

Biguanides
Metformin

- Oral therapy
- Exact mechanism unknown
- Primary effect: ↓ **hepatic glucose production**
  - Inhibits gluconeogenesis

Biguanides
Metformin

- Lowers serum **free fatty acids**
  - ↓ substrates for gluconeogenesis
  - ↓ triglycerides
  - Small ↓ LDL
  - Small ↑ HDL

Biguanides
Metformin

- Other effects
  - Reduced glucose absorption from GI tract
  - Direct stimulation of glycolysis in tissues → ↑ glucose uptake
  - Reduced glucagon levels
- Leads to ↑ **insulin effect** (insulin sensitivity)
  - Insulin levels fall slightly on therapy

Biguanides
Metformin

- Usually **1st line in type 2 diabetes**
  - Associated with **weight loss**
  - Rarely causes hypoglycemia (unlike insulin/sulfonylureas)
- Does not depend on beta cells
  - Can be given to patients with advanced diabetes

Biguanides
Metformin

- Most common adverse effect is **GI upset**
  - Nausea, abdominal pain
  - Can cause a metallic taste in the mouth

Biguanides
Metformin

- Rarely can cause **lactic acidosis**
  - Exact mechanism unclear/controversial
  - Metformin can increase conversion of glucose to lactate
  - Beneficial for lowering glucose levels
  - Too much → lactic acidosis
  - Can be life threatening

Metformin
Lactic Acidosis

- Almost always occurs associated with:
  - **Renal insufficiency**
  - Liver disease or alcohol abuse
  - Acute heart failure
  - Hypoxia
  - Serious acute illness
- Metformin not used in patients with low GFR
- Often "held" when patients acutely ill
- Also held during IV contrast tests

Sulfonylureas

- Bind to sulfonylurea receptor in pancreas
  - Associated with ATP-dependent K+ channel in beta cells
- Sulfonylureas close **K+ channels** in beta cells
  - Changes resting potential
  - Results in depolarization (Ca influx)
- More sensitive to glucose/amino acids
- ↑ insulin release ("insulin secretagogues")

H_2N ⎯ C(=O) ⎯ NH_2
Urea

Sulfonylurea

Sulfonylureas

- Oral drugs
- Each generation more potent
- ↓ dosage used → ↓ side effects
- First generation
  - Tolbutamide, Chlorpropamide, Tolazamide
- Second generation
  - Glyburide, glipizide
- 3rd generation: Glimepiride

Sulfonylureas
Adverse Effects

- **Hypoglycemia** is the most common side effect
  - Glucagon levels fall (unclear mechanism)
  - May occur with exercise or skipping meals

Sulfonylureas
Adverse Effects

- Can also cause **weight gain**
  - More insulin release
  - Insulin causes weight gain

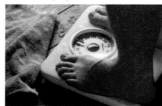

Wikipedia/Public Domain

Sulfonylureas
Adverse Effects

- Chlorpropamide
  - **Flushing** with alcohol consumption
    - Inhibits acetaldehyde dehydrogenase (disulfiram)
  - Hyponatremia (↑ADH activity)

Meglitinides
Repaglinide, Nateglinide

- Oral therapy
- Different chemical structure from sulfonylureas
- Similar mechanism
- Close K+ channels in beta cells → ↑ insulin secretion
- Short acting
- Given **prior to meals**
- Major side effect is hypoglycemia
- No sulfur → can be used in **sulfa allergy**

Thiazolidinediones (TZDs)
Pioglitazone, Rosiglitazone

- Oral therapy
- **Decreases insulin resistance**

Thiazolidinediones (TZDs)
Pioglitazone, Rosiglitazone

- Act on **PPAR-γ receptors**
  - Nuclear receptor
  - Highest levels in **adipose tissue**
  - Also found in muscle, liver, other tissues
  - Modulate expression of genes
- TZDs bind PPAR-gamma
- TZD-PPAR bind **retinoid X receptors** (RXR)
- Complex modifies gene transcription

> NOTE: Fibrates activate PPAR-α
> Lower triglycerides

Thiazolidinediones
Potential mechanisms

- **GLUT-4**
  - Glucose transporter
  - Transcription upregulated
- **Adiponectin**
  - Adipocyte secretory protein
  - ↑ **insulin sensitivity** via several mechanisms
  - Signaling may lead to improved glucose levels
- Antagonism of **TNF alpha** insulin resistance
  - TNF-α levels fall

Thiazolidinediones
Adverse Effects

- **Weight gain**
  - May cause proliferation of adipocytes
  - Also lead to fluid retention
- Risk of hepatotoxicity
  - Troglitazone removed from market due to liver failure

Thiazolidinediones
Adverse Effects

- Edema
  - Occurs in ~5% patients
  - Due to PPAR-γ effects in nephron → ↑ Na retention
  - Risk of **pulmonary edema**
  - Not used in patients with **advanced heart failure**

Glucosidase Inhibitors
Acarbose, Miglitol, Voglibose

- **Competitive inhibitors of intestinal α-glucosidases**
  - Sucrase, maltase, glucoamylase, dextranase
  - Enzymes of brush border of intestinal cells
  - Hydrolyze starches, oligosaccharides, disaccharides
- Slows absorption of glucose
  - Less absorption upper small intestine
  - More in distal small intestine

Glucosidase Inhibitors
Acarbose, Miglitol, Voglibose

- Taken orally before meals
- **Less spike in glucose after meals**
- Lowers mean glucose level → lowers A1c
- Less insulin used ("insulin sparing")
- Main side effect: **GI upset**
  - Flatulence
  - Diarrhea

Amylin Analogs
Pramlintide

- Amylin: protein stored in beta cells
- Co-secreted with insulin
- Several effects (mechanisms poorly understood)
  - Suppresses glucagon release
  - Delays gastric emptying
  - Reduces appetite
- Allows insulin to work more effectively

Amylin Analogs
Pramlintide

- Given SQ with meals
- Always given with insulin (type I or type 2)
- **Hypoglycemia** may result → need to ↓ insulin dose
- Can also cause nausea

Incretins

- Hormones that ↑ **insulin secretion**
- GIP (glucose-dependent insulinotropic peptide)
  - Produced by K cells of small intestine
- **GLP-1 (glucagon-like peptide-1)**
  - Produced by L-cells of small intestine
  - Secreted after meals
  - Stimulates insulin release (similar to GIP)
  - Also blunts glucagon release, slows gastric emptying
- Oral glucose metabolized faster than IV glucose

GLP-1 Analogs
Exenatide, Liraglutide

- Exenatide: Usually given SQ prior to meals
  - Once weekly version available
- Liraglutide: SQ once daily
- GI side effects: nausea, vomiting, diarrhea

DPP-4 Inhibitors
Sitagliptin, Linagliptin

- DPP-4: Dipeptidyl peptidase 4
  - Enzyme expressed on many cells
  - Inhibits release of GIP and GLP-1
- Inhibition → ↑ GLP-1
- Oral drugs, once a day
- Side effects: **Infections**
  - Reports of urinary and respiratory infections

SGLT2 Inhibitors
Canagliflozin, Dapagliflozin

- SGLT2
  - Expressed in proximal tubule
  - Reabsorbs ~90% percent filtered glucose
- Inhibition → loss of glucose in urine
  - Lowers glucose levels
  - Also causes mild osmotic diuresis

Proximal Tubule

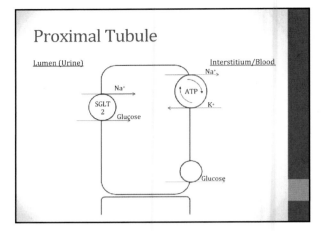

SGLT2 Inhibitors
Canagliflozin, Dapagliflozin

- Oral drugs taken once daily
- Lead to mild weight loss
- May improve outcomes in heart failure
- Adverse effects
  - Vulvovaginal candidiasis
  - UTIs
- Not recommended with advanced renal disease

Diabetes Therapy
Helpful Tips

- Renal failure: Avoid **metformin** (lactic acidosis)
- Advanced heart failure
  - Avoid **TZDs** (fluid retention)
  - Avoid **metformin** (lactic acidosis)
- Insulin generally safe with any comorbidity

Reproductive Hormones

Jason Ryan, MD, MPH

Reproductive Hormones

- **Estrogens** and **androgens**
- Development and function of sex organs
- Secondary sexual characteristics (puberty)

Estrogens

Potency
Estradiol> Estrone > Estriol

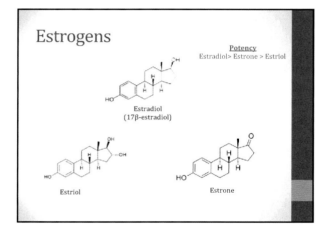

Estradiol
(17β-estradiol)

Estriol

Estrone

Androgens

Potency
DHT > Testosterone > others

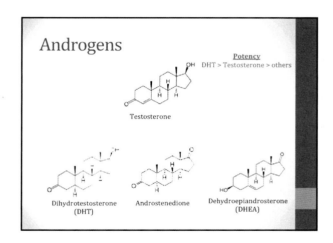

Testosterone

Dihydrotestosterone
(DHT)

Androstenedione

Dehydroepiandrosterone
(DHEA)

Reproductive Hormones

- **Steroid hormones** (from **cholesterol**)
- Poorly soluble in plasma
- Carried by **sex hormone binding globulins** (SHBGs)
  - Smaller amount by albumin
- Cross lipid bilayer of cells
- Bind to **intracellular receptors**

SHBG
Sex Hormone Binding Globulins

- Glycoproteins
- Produced by the **liver**
- Binds androgens more than estrogens

$$A > E$$

65

Estrogen Amplification

- Free hormones → clinical effects
- ↑ SHBG → ↓ free androgens and estrogens
  - More effect on androgens
  - ↑ ratio estrogens to androgens
- "Amplification" of estrogen effects

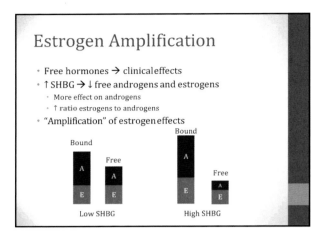

SHBG
Sex Hormone Binding Globulins

Causes	↑SHBG	↓SHBG
Causes	Estrogens Hyperthyroidism	Androgens Hypothyroidism Nephrotic Syndrome
Hormones	↑ Estrogen effects	↑ Androgen effects
Clinical Effects	Gynecomastia (men)	Hirsutism (women)

Cirrhosis

- ↑ estrogen effects
  - Gynecomastia
  - Spider nevi
  - Palmar erythema
  - Testicular atrophy
  - Impotence
- Altered metabolism/excretion → ↑ estrogen
- ↑ SHBG → ↑ estrogen effects
- Clinical features of ↑estrogens/↓androgens

Reproductive Hormones

- Hypothalamus: GnRH
- Pituitary:
  - Follicle stimulating hormone
  - Luteinizing Hormone
- Testes/Ovaries
- Androgens/estrogens

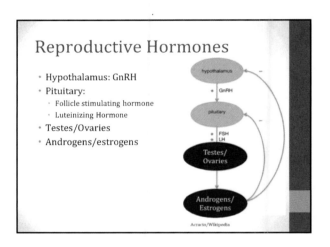

Puberty

- FSH and LH are low before puberty
- Rise at puberty in boys and girls

GNRH
Gonadotropin-releasing hormone

- Peptide produced by hypothalamus
- Released in pulses ("pulsatile")
  - Frequency and amplitude of pulses varies
  - Changes effect release of LH/FSH from pituitary

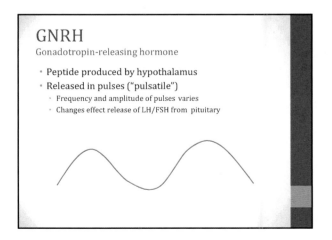

GNRH
Gonadotropin-releasing hormone

- **Gq protein system with IP3 second messenger**
  - PIP2 = Phosphatidylinositol bisphosphate
  - IP3 = Inositol trisphosphate
  - DAG = Diacylglycerol

Eak435s /Wikipedia

Leuprolide

- GnRH agonists
  - Derived from GnRH
  - **D-amino acid substitution** for native L-amino acid
  - Resistant to degradation
  - ↑ half-life → occupies receptors for prolonged period of time

Leuprolide

- Initial binding can stimulate LH/FSH release
- Chronic treatment → ↓LH/FSH
  - Down-regulation of GnRH receptor
  - Pituitary desensitization
- Suppresses ovarian follicular growth and ovulation
- Low levels of estradiol and progesterone
  - Similar to menopause

Leuprolide
Uses

- Pulsatile (rarely done)
  - Stimulation of LH/FSH release
  - Administered by infusion pump
  - Dose varies about every 90 minutes
  - Used to create LH surge for ovulation (infertility)

Leuprolide
Uses

- Continuous
  - Suppression of LH/FSH release
  - Endometriosis
  - Uterine fibroids (leiomyomata)
  - Prostate cancer
  - Precocious puberty

Kallmann Syndrome

- **Absence of GnRH** secretion from hypothalamus
- Impaired migration of GnRH neurons from origin in **olfactory bulb** to hypothalamus
- Almost always occurs in males (5:1 ratio)
- Key features: hypogonadism and **anosmia**
- **Low GnRH/FSH/LH/Testosterone**
- Delayed puberty
- Small testes

Pituitary Reproductive Hormones

- LH, FSH
- Proteins
- LH, FSH, TSH and HCG are "heterodimers"
  - Dimer = two molecules; hetero = different
- Two chains: α and β
- Same α, different β

Pituitary Hormones

- All have a cAMP second messenger system

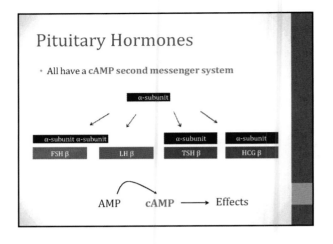

Male Reproductive Hormones

Jason Ryan, MD, MPH

Male Reproductive System

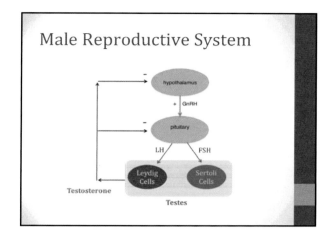

Leydig Cell

Adrenal Cortex
DHEA
Androstenedione
Testosterone

Cholesterol

Dehydroepiandrosterone (DHEA)

Androstenedione

Testosterone

Dihydrotestosterone
DHT

- Testosterone **converted to DHT** in peripheral tissues
- Enzymes: **5-α reductase**
- Many testosterone effects mediated by DHT
- DHT: ↑ potency
  - Binds androgen receptor > testosterone
  - More stable

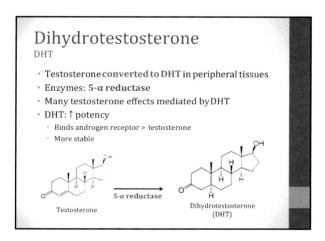

Testosterone   5-α reductase   Dihydrotestosterone (DHT)

Finasteride

- 5-α reductase inhibited by finasteride
- Used for treatment of **prostatic hyperplasia**
- Also used to treat **hair loss** in men

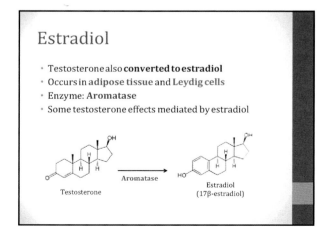

Testosterone   Finasteride X   5-α reductase   Dihydrotestosterone (DHT)

Estradiol

- Testosterone also **converted to estradiol**
- Occurs in **adipose tissue** and **Leydig cells**
- Enzyme: **Aromatase**
- Some testosterone effects mediated by estradiol

Testosterone   Aromatase   Estradiol (17β-estradiol)

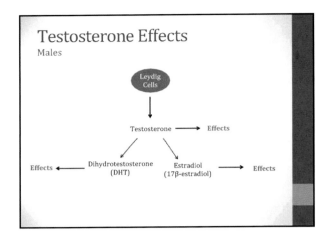

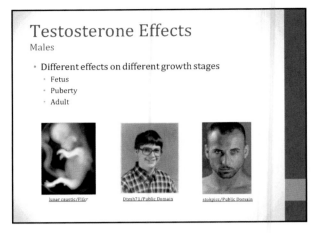

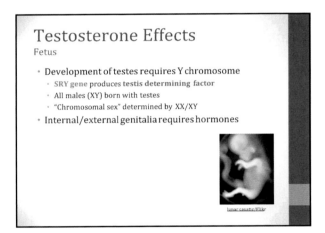

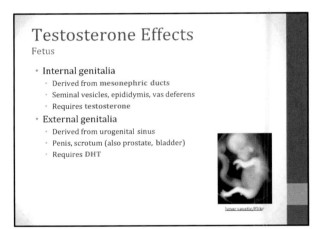

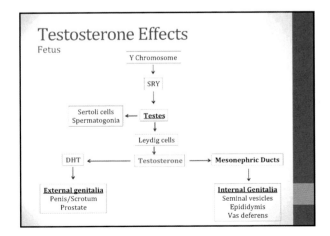

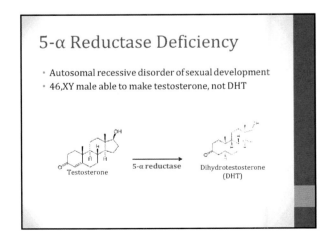

5-α Reductase Deficiency

- **Normal internal genitalia**
  - Normal epididymis, vas deferens, seminal vesicles
  - Empty into a blind-ending vagina
- External genitalia predominately female
  - Absent external male genitalia
  - Range of female genitalia seen +/- hypospadius
  - Sometimes diagnosed at birth due to ambiguous genitalia

5-α Reductase Deficiency

- Typical case
  - Male with ambiguous genitalia
  - Female child with masculinization at puberty
  - Blind vagina
  - Absence of uterus
  - Bilateral undescended testes
  - Normal testosterone levels

Testosterone Effects
Puberty

Dtesh71/Public Domain

- Enlargement of the scrotum, and testes
- Increased penis size
- Enlargement of seminal vesicles/prostate
- Growth of pubic hair
- Hair on face/underarms
- Deepening of voice

Testosterone Effects
Puberty

- Growth spurt (**via estrogens**)
  - Increased linear growth
  - Closure of epiphyseal plates

Acne

Wikipedia/Public Domain

- Associated with increased sebum
  - Secretion of **sebaceous glands**
- Androgen receptors on sebaceous glands
  - Androgens stimulate growth/secretions
- Acne common in puberty
- Also common in other forms androgen excess
  - Polycystic ovarian syndrome
  - Congenital adrenal hyperplasia

Testosterone Effects
Adults

- Prostate growth
  - Finasteride → ↓DHT → Treatment of BPH
  - Testosterone therapy → BPH
- May effect lipids
  - Exogenous testosterone → ↓ HDL/↑ LDL
- Male pattern balding

Androgenic Alopecia
"Male Pattern Balding"

- Most common type of hair loss in men
- Anterior scalp, mid scalp, temporal scalp, and vertex
- Caused by **androgens**
  - Occurs after puberty
  - Will not occur with androgen deficiency
- **DHT** is key androgen
  - Responds to finasteride treatment

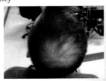

Welshsk/Wikipedia

Male Hypogonadism

- Many congenital and acquired causes
- May occur with **aging**
  - ↓ serum testosterone
  - ↑ sex hormone-binding globulin (SHBG)
  - ↓ serum free testosterone
- May be associated with:
  - ↓ sexual function
  - ↓ bone mass
  - Anemia
- Limited data on hormone replacement for decreased testosterone due to aging

Testosterone Therapy

- Used in male hypogonadism
- Results in:
  - Increased muscle mass
  - Increased bone density
- Potential adverse effects
  - ↑ hematocrit
  - Acne
  - Balding
  - Worsening BPH

Spermatogenesis

- Suppressed by exogenous testosterone
- Testosterone suppresses LH secretion
- ↓ testosterone from Leydig cells
- Exogenous hormone weak activity in testes
- ↓ **spermatogenesis**

Anabolic Steroids

- **High dosages** of androgens used by body builders
  - Exogenous testosterone
  - Androgen precursors
- All lead to ↑ testosterone effects → ↑ muscle mass
- Adverse effects
  - ↓ HDL/↑ LDL
  - Erythrocytosis
  - Small testes (suppression of FSH/LH)
  - Azoospermia
  - Gynecomastia (↑conversion to estradiol)

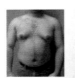

Image courtesy Dr. Mordcai Blau/Wikipedia

Spironolactone

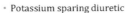
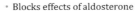

Spironolactone

- Potassium sparing diuretic
- Blocks effects of aldosterone
- Used in hypertension, heart failure
- Key side effect: **gynecomastia** (~10%)
  - Blocks androgen receptor
  - ↓ androgen production from androstenedione
- Result:
  - ↑ **estrogen effects**
  - ↓ **androgen effects**

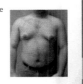

Image courtesy Dr. Mordcai Blau/Wikipedia

Spironolactone

- **Acne, hirsutism, alopecia** in women
  - Blunts testosterone effects
  - Enhances estrogen effects
- Amenorrhea
  - Stimulates progesterone receptors

Spironolactone

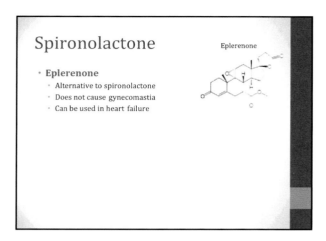

Spironolactone

- **Eplerenone**
  - Alternative to spironolactone
  - Does not cause gynecomastia
  - Can be used in heart failure

Eplerenone

Sertoli Cells

- Support and nourish developing spermatozoa
- Regulate spermatogenesis

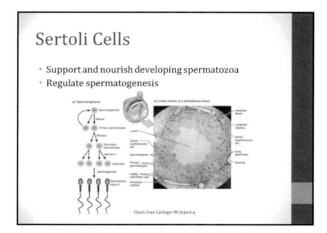

Sertoli Cells

- Stimulated by FSH
- Supported by Leydig cell testosterone (paracrine)
- Need **FSH and LH** for normal spermatogenesis

Sertoli Cells

- Form **blood-testis barrier**
- Tight junctions between adjacent Sertoli cells
- Isolates sperm
- Protection from autoimmune attack

Sertoli Cells

- Secrete **inhibin B**: Inhibits FSH

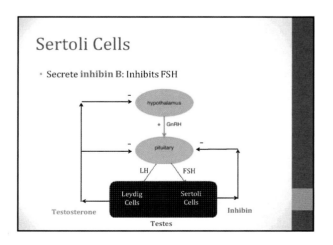

Sertoli Cells

- Secrete **androgen-binding protein (ABP)**
  - Raises/maintains local testosterone levels
  - Intra-testicular testosterone concentration 100x peripheral
- Produce **anti-mullerian hormone**
  - Results in degeneration of mullerian ducts

Anti-mullerian Hormone

- In utero (XX or XY): **Two systems**
  - Indifferent gonad (can develop into ovaries or testes)
  - Paramesonephric (Mullerian) duct: female structure
  - Mesonephric (Wolffian) duct: male structures
- Y chromosome → testes → Sertoli cells
- Secretion of **anti-mullerian hormone**
  - Mullerian inhibitory hormone/substance
- Degeneration of mullerian system
- Leaves gonad and mesonephric ducts

Male Development

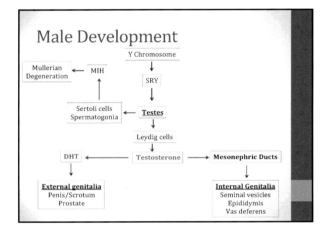

CAIS
Complete Androgen Insensitivity Syndrome

- Mutation of androgen receptor in males (XY)
- No ovaries; testes form in utero (SRY gene)
- No cellular response to androgens
  - No internal or external male genital development
- Sertoli cells (testes) present → MIH
  - Degeneration of mullerian structures
  - Absent uterus, fallopian tubes

CAIS
Complete Androgen Insensitivity Syndrome

- At puberty:
  - Breasts develop (testosterone → estrogen)
  - No armpit/pubic hair (depends on androgens)
- Amenorrhea (no uterus)
- Abdominal testes

Disorders of Sex Development

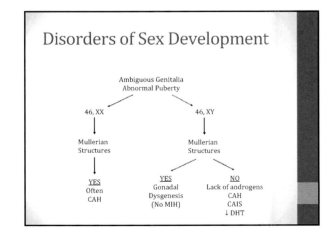

Temperature Effects

- Spermatogenesis requires ↓temperature
- Sertoli cells sensitive to temperature
  - ↓spermatogenesis with higher temperature
  - ↓inhibin production with higher temperature (↑FSH)
- Leydig cells less sensitive
  - Testosterone production usually maintained higher temps

Cryptorchidism

- "Hidden testes"
- Usually due to undescended testes
  - Abdominal
  - Inguinal canal
- Can be unilateral/bilateral

Cryptorchidism
Complications

- Low sperm counts
  - ↑temperature effects on Sertoli cells
  - Low inhibin levels
- ↑risk of germ cell tumors
- Inguinal hernias
- Testicular torsion
  - Testicle rotates → twists spermatic cord
  - Compression of veins → ↓blood flow
  - Hemorrhagic infarction

Cryptorchidism
Treatment

- Testes may descend on their own
  - Usually occurs by 6 months of age
- Orchiopexy
  - Surgical placement of the testis in scrotum
  - Sperm counts usually become normal
  - Done after 6 months of age

Bilateral Undescended Testes

- Phenotypical male with bilateral non-palpable testes
- Dangerous cause: congenital adrenal hyperplasia
  - Female (XX) exposed to increased androgens
  - Ambiguous genitalia may appear male with absent testes
  - Risk of shock from low cortisol
  - Key tests: ACTH, Cortisol
- Testes may be absent
  - Agenesis or atrophy (intrauterine vascular compromise)
  - Serum testing often done
  - Absent testes: ↑LH/FSH, absence of MIH

Varicocele

- Dilatation of pampiniform plexus of spermatic veins

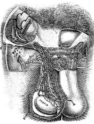

Wikipedia/Public Domain

Varicocele

- Caused by obstruction to outflow of venous blood
- More common on **left**
  - Left spermatic vein → left renal (long course)
  - Compressed between aorta and superior mesenteric artery
  - "Nutcracker effect"
  - Right vein drains directly to IVC
- Associated with renal cell carcinoma
  - Invades renal vein

Varicocele

- Scrotal pain and swelling
  - "Bag of worms"
- More swelling with:
  - Valsalva
  - Standing
- Diagnosed by **ultrasound**
- Can cause infertility
  - ↑ temperature
  - Poor blood flow

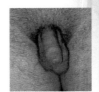

Fisch12/Wikipedia

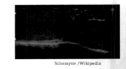

Schomynv /Wikipedia

Varicocele
Treatment

- Surgery (varicocelectomy)
  - Isolate dilated/abnormal veins
  - Redirect blood flow to normal veins
- Embolization
  - Interventional radiology procedure
  - Catheter inserted into dilated/abnormal veins
  - Coil or sclerosants used to clot off veins

Female Reproductive Hormones

Jason Ryan, MD, MPH

Estrogens

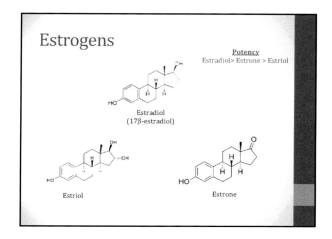

Potency
Estradiol > Estrone > Estriol

Estradiol
(17β-estradiol)

Estriol

Estrone

Ovarian Follicle

- Egg surrounded by cells
- Two key cell types: **theca and granulosa** cells

Antrum
(fluid)

Granulosa
Cells

Theca
Cells

Oocyte

Hormone Synthesis
Estrogens

- **Theca cells**
  - Convert cholesterol into androstenedione
  - Stimulated by LH (via cAMP 2nd messenger)
- **Granulosa cells**
  - Convert androstenedione into estradiol
  - Stimulated by FSH (via cAMP 2nd messenger)
  - Also produce inhibin → suppresses FSH

Hormone Synthesis
Estrogens

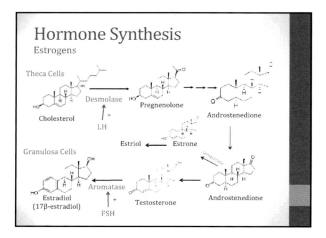

Theca Cells

Cholesterol — Desmolase → Pregnenolone —→ —→ Androstenedione

LH +

Granulosa Cells

Estradiol
(17β-estradiol)

Estriol ← Estrone

Aromatase +

FSH

Testosterone ← Androstenedione

Female Reproductive System

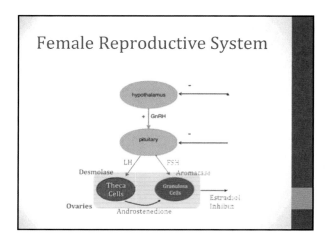

hypothalamus

+ GnRH

pituitary

LH   FSH

Desmolase   Aromatase

Theca
Cells

Granulosa
Cells

Ovaries   Androstenedione

Estradiol
Inhibin

Estrogen Effects

- Growth of follicle
  - Theca/Granulosa cells → estradiol → follicular growth
- Increase SHBG
  - Amplifies estrogen effects
- Lipids
  - Raises HDL
  - Lowers LDL

Estrogen Effects
Puberty

- Breast enlargement
- Pigmentation of areolas
  - Also seen in pregnancy
- Female body habitus
  - Narrow shoulders, broad hips
  - Female fat distribution in breasts and buttocks
- Note: Pubic and axillary hair from androgens

Estrogen Effects
Pituitary

- ↓ FSH secretion (negative feedback)
- ↓ LH secretion (negative feedback)
- Exception: Can trigger LH surge (positive feedback)

Progesterone

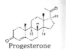
Progesterone

- Synthesized by corpus luteum
  - Also placenta, adrenal glands, testes
- Most bound to albumin
- Short half life → metabolized by liver
- Main target is uterus, cervix, vagina

Progesterone Effects

- Many effects oppose estrogen
  - Decreases expression estrogen receptors
- Many effects favorable to pregnancy

Progesterone Effects

- Secretory phase of uterine cycle
- Thickens cervical mucous
  - Prevents sperm entry
- Prevents uterine contractions
  - ↓ uterine excitability
  - ↑ membrane potential of uterine smooth muscle
  - Uterine smooth muscle relaxation
- Raises body temperature (seen in pregnancy)
- Inhibits LH/FSH release

Oral Contraceptives

- Analogs of estrogens and progesterone
  - "Estrogens and progestins"
- Progestin only
  - Oral "mini pill"
  - Medroxyprogesterone injection (Depo-Provera)
- Combination pills
  - Contain estrogen and progesterone

Oral Contraceptives

Progesterone

Estradiol

Norethisterone

Ethinyl estradiol

Progestin Only

- Suppress ovulation via negative feedback on FSH/LH
- Thickens cervical mucus
  - Obstructs sperm
  - May protect against PID
- Thins endometrium
  - Prevents implantation

Progestin Only

- Disadvantages
  - Same time every day (+/- 3 hours)
  - Irregular bleeding, spotting
- Advantages
  - No estrogen risks/side effects

Medroxyprogesterone
Depo-Provera

- Injectable, progestin-only contraceptive
- Intramuscular or subcutaneous
- Once every 3 months

Combination OCPs

- Combination of progestin and estrogen
- Better suppression of follicular growth
  - Progesterone suppresses LH
  - Estrogen suppresses FSH
- Estrogen stabilizes endothelium
  - Less breakthrough bleeding
- Estrogen increases effect of progesterone
  - More progesterone receptors

Combination OCP Risks

- Breakthrough bleeding
  - Most common side effect
  - More frequent if low estrogen component
- Hypertension (usually mild)

Combination OCP Risks

- **Thrombosis**
  - Estrogen increases clotting factors
  - Usually venous thrombosis: DVT/PE
  - Rarely arterial thrombosis: stroke/MI
- Cancer
  - Conflicting data
  - May ↓ risk of endometrial and ovarian cancer
  - May ↑ risk breast, cervical, liver cancer

Combination OCPs
Contraindications

- **Smokers** >35 years of age
  - Risk of CV events
- History of DVT/PE

Pixabay/Public Domain

80

Menstrual Cycle

Jason Ryan, MD, MPH

Female Reproductive System

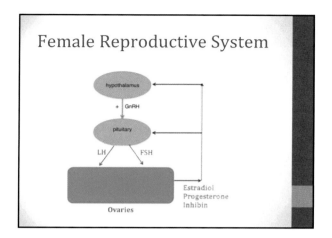

Ovaries
Basic Principles

- Contain **follicles**
  - Spherical collection of cells
  - Contains a single oocyte
- Each menstrual cycle one egg matures/releases

Ovarian Follicle

- Egg surrounded by cells
- Two key cell types: **theca and granulosa** cells

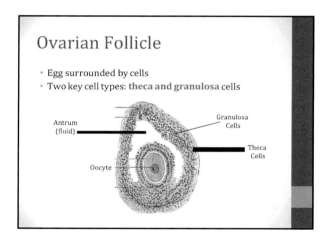

Ovarian Follicle

- During menstrual cycle, follicles mature
- One "dominant" follicle will release egg

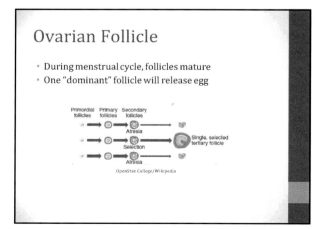

Menstrual Cycle
Basic Principles

- Phases
  - Follicular (growth of follicles)
  - Ovulation
  - Luteal (preparation for pregnancy)

Menstrual Cycle

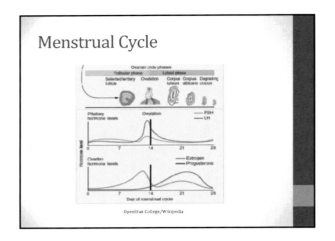

OpenStax College/Wikipedia

Menstrual Cycle
Follicular phase

- ↑ GnRH pulse frequency
- ↑ FSH → ↑ estradiol production from ovaries
- Recruitment of follicles
- ↑ estradiol → ↓ FSH/LH (negative feedback)
- Selection of one dominant/ovulatory follicle
- 10-14 days (varies in length)

Menstrual Cycle
Ovulation

- **Mid-cycle surge**
  - Switch from negative feedback to positive feedback
  - Estradiol triggers ↑ frequency GnRH pules → **LH surge**
  - Oocyte released from follicle ~36 hours after LH surge
- **Basis for ovulation testing**
  - Urine detection of LH

OTRS/Wikipedia

Mittelschmerz

- Mid-cycle pain
- Due to:
  - Enlargement of follicle or follicular rupture with bleeding
- Usually **mild, unilateral pain**
- Usually resolves in hours to days
- Can mimic other disorders (**appendicitis**)

Menstrual Cycle
Luteal phase

- **Corpus luteum forms**
  - Temporary endocrine gland formed from follicle
  - Produces large amounts of **progesterone**
  - Also some estradiol
- **Progesterone/estradiol → ↓LH/FSH**
  - Negative feedback

Menstrual Cycle
Luteal phase

- Eventually corpus luteum degrades
- ↓ progesterone → menstruation
  - Occurs 14 days after ovulation
- If fertilization occurs:
  - Embryo makes **human chorionic gonadotropin (hCG)**
  - Maintains the corpus luteum and progesterone production
  - Progesterone maintains suppression of LH/FSH

Uterine Cycle

- Changes in **endometrium**
- Driven by estrogens and progesterone
- Parallels ovarian cycle
- Two phases:
  - Proliferative phase = follicular phase of ovary
  - Secretory phase = luteal phase of ovary

Uterine Cycle
Proliferative Phase

- Menstruation followed by endometrial **proliferation**
- Stimulated by **estrogen**
- Endometrial thickness increases (>10x)
- Growth of glands, stroma, blood vessels

Uterine Cycle
Secretory Phase

- Occurs **after ovulation**
- **Progesterone** inhibits proliferation of endometrium
- Numerous secretions released to **prepare for embryo**
- Changes in blood vessels
  - Vessels grow and coil
  - Form "**spiral arteries**" about 9th postovulatory day
  - Critical for implantation, support of fertilized egg

Menstruation

- Progesterone levels fall
- Vasoconstriction of spiral arteries
- **Apoptosis** of endometrial cells occurs
- Collapse and desquamation of endometrium

Menstrual and Uterine Cycles

Amenorrhea

- Primary amenorrhea
  - Failure of menses at puberty
  - Usually anatomic or genetic abnormality
- Secondary amenorrhea
  - Cessation of normal menses after prior normal periods

Progestin Challenge

- Older test for causes of amenorrhea
- Many false positives
- Administration of progestin (oral or IM)
- Observation of menstrual bleeding within 7 days

Progestin Challenge

- Bleeding
  - Indicates estrogen is present
  - Suggests anovulation
  - Corpus luteum not forming (inadequate progesterone)
  - Classic cause: **PCOS**
- No bleeding
  - Suggests estrogen not present (ovarian dysfunction)
  - Or menstrual outflow problem
  - Can follow-up with estrogen-progestin challenge
  - Common cause: **Menopause**

Mullerian Dysgenesis

- Cause of primary amenorrhea
- Failure of **Mullerian duct** development
- Absent upper vagina and/or uterus
- Ovaries normal
- Estrogen/progesterone levels normal
- Normal LH/FSH levels

Secondary Amenorrhea

- Most common cause: **pregnancy**
  - Screen with HCG measurement
- Thyroid disease (hypo/hyper)
- Prolactinoma
  - Inhibition of GnRH release → ↓ LH/FSH
- Cushing syndrome

Secondary Amenorrhea

- **Low body weight**
  - "Functional hypothalamic amenorrhea"
  - Stress plus low caloric intake → ↓ GnRH/LH/FSH
  - Can occur in anorexia

Menopause

- Permanent cessation of menstrual periods
- Cause by **depletion of ovarian follicles**
- Median age = 51 years
- Usually preceded by abnormal periods

Menopause

- Loss of estradiol production from ovaries
  - Source of estrogen becomes adipose tissue
  - Aromatase coverts androstenedione to **estrone**
- Also loss of inhibin production from follicles
  - Inhibin normally suppresses FSH release
  - ↑↑ FSH is an early finding approaching menopause
- Eventually FSH and LH levels both elevated

Androstenedione → Aromatase → Estrone

Menopause
Symptoms

- **Hot flashes**
  - Subjective sensation of warmth
  - Usually lasts a few minutes and passes
  - Associated with drop in estrogen levels
  - Can be treated with hormone replacement
- Vaginal atrophy
  - Thin, dry, friable
  - Loss of estrogen stimulation

Menopause
Symptoms

- Osteoporosis
  - Bone loss from lack of estrogen
- Cardiovascular disease
  - Risk increases after menopause
  - May be due in part due to estrogen deficiency

HRT
Hormone Replacement Therapy

- Oral or transdermal estradiol
- Progestin added in women with intact uterus
  - Prevents endometrial hyperplasia

HRT
Hormone Replacement Therapy

- Benefits:
  - **Relieves hot flashes**
  - Improves bone density
- Possible risks:
  - ↑ risk of DVT/Stroke/MI
  - ↑ risk of breast cancer

PCOS
Polycystic Ovarian Syndrome

- Common cause secondary amenorrhea
- Genetics plus diet/obesity → ↑ LH:FSH ratio
- LH drives androstenedione from theca cells
- Some androgens → estrone in adipose tissue
- Estrone → ↓ FSH → anovulation

PCOS

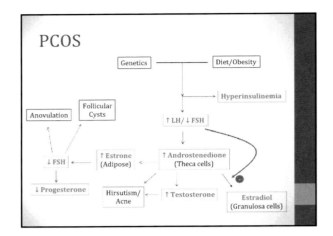

Genetics — Diet/Obesity

Hyperinsulinemia

↑ LH/ ↓ FSH

Anovulation | Follicular Cysts

↓ FSH | ↑ Estrone (Adipose) ← ↑ Androstenedione (Theca cells)

↓ Progesterone | Hirsutism/ Acne ← ↑ Testosterone | Estradiol (Granulosa cells)

PCOS
Clinical features

- Occurs in obese females
- **Hirsutism** (facial hair)
- Acne
- Amenorrhea
- **Infertility**
- Ultrasound: multiple follicular cysts

Hyperinsulinemia

- PCOS associated with insulin resistance
- More than expected for degree of obesity
- Can lead to diabetes

PCOS
Diagnosis

- Usually diagnosed clinically
- Can measure **total testosterone**
- LH and FSH may be within normal range
  - But LH:FSH ratio usually > 2:1 or 3:1

PCOS
Treatment

- **Weight loss**
- **Oral contraceptives**
  - Suppress LH
  - Estrogen → ↑ SHBG → ↓ androgens
- **Spironolactone**
  - Blocks androgens
- **Metformin/TZDs**
  - Diabetes drugs that improves insulin resistance
  - Not routinely used unless patient develops diabetes

PCOS
Other Features

- Risk of **diabetes**
  - ~10% of women with PCOS develop DM by 40 years old
- **Acanthosis Nigricans**
  - Plaques of darkened skin
  - Associated with insulin resistance
  - Common in diabetes, PCOS, also gastric cancer
- **Endometrial cancer**
  - Unopposed estrogen (lack of progesterone)
  - ↑ risk of endometrial hyperplasia and carcinoma

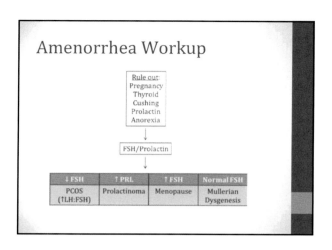

Pituitary Gland

Jason Ryan, MD, MPH

Pituitary Gland

- "Master gland"
- Endocrine gland at base of brain
- Sits in small cavity of sphenoid bone: sella turcica

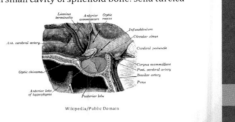

Wikipedia/Public Domain

Pituitary Gland

- Connected to **hypothalamus** via pituitary stalk
- Connects to **median eminence** of hypothalamus
  - One of the circumventricular organs (CVOs)
  - Does not contain blood brain barrier

Posterior Pituitary Gland
Neurohypophysis

- Secretes ADH (vasopressin) and oxytocin
- Derived from **neural ectoderm** in floor of forebrain
- Contains axons and nerve terminals
- Neurons originate in hypothalamus
- **Paraventricular and supraoptic nuclei**
  - Paraventricular: Oxytocin
  - Supraoptic: ADH

Anterior Pituitary Gland
Adenohypophysis

- Derived from **Rathke's pouch**
  - Outgrowth of oral cavity
- Contains five cell types that make hormones

Cell Type	Hormone
Corticotrophs	Adrenocorticotropic hormone (ACTH)
Thyrotrophs	Thyroid-stimulating hormone (TSH)
Gonadotrophs	Luteinizing hormone (LH) Follicle-stimulating hormone (FSH)
Somatotrophs	Growth hormone (GH)
Lactotrophs	Prolactin

Hypothalamic Portal System

- Main blood supply to anterior pituitary gland
- Delivers releasing/inhibiting hormones

Hypothalamus	Pituitary
Corticotropin-releasing hormone (CRH)	ACTH
Thyrotropin-releasing hormone (TRH)	TSH
Gonadotropin-releasing hormone (GnRH)	LH/FSH
Growth hormone–releasing hormone (GHRH)	GH
Dopamine	Prolactin
Somatostatin	GH, TSH

Prolactin

- Protein hormone
- Regulates milk production in mothers

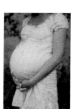

Øyvind Holmstad/Wikipedia

Prolactin

- Under **inhibitory control** from hypothalamus
  - Hypothalamus releases **dopamine**
  - Inhibits lactotrophs via binding to D2 receptors
  - Destruction of hypothalamus: ↑ prolactin
- Prolactin feedback on hypothalamus
  - Increases dopamine release → ↓ prolactin

Prolactin

- Many other substances affect prolactin release
  - VIP, Oxytocin, TRH, others
- **TRH** (thyrotropin-releasing hormone)
  - Elevated in hypothyroidism
  - Hypothyroidism predisposes to hyperprolactinemia
- Hypothyroidism in differential for:
  - Pituitary enlargement
  - Hyperprolactinemia

Prolactin in Pregnancy

- **Estrogen** stimulates prolactin release
  - Stimulates gene transcription
  - Stimulates release from lactotrophs
- Marked increase in lactotrophs during pregnancy
- Pituitary can grow in size

Prolactin in Pregnancy

- Prolactin **inhibits GnRH release**
- Results in cessation of ovulation/menstruation

Prolactin in Pregnancy

- Prolactin stimulates growth of mammary glands
- Milk production in pregnancy does not occur
  - **Estradiol and progesterone** block prolactin effect on milk
- After childbirth → ↓ estradiol and progesterone
  - Milk production occurs

Dopamine Agonists
Cabergoline, Bromocriptine

- Can be used to treat Parkinson's disease
- Also used to treat prolactinomas
- Will **inhibit prolactin release** (via D2 receptors)

Pituitary Adenomas

- Tumors of any cell type of anterior pituitary
- May result in increased secretion of hormones
- Most common secreting tumor: **prolactinoma**

Cell Type	Disease
Lactotrophs	Hyperprolactinemia
Thyrotrophs	Central hyperthyroidism
Corticotrophs	Cushing's disease
Somatotrophs	Acromegaly/Gigantism

Pituitary Adenomas
General Symptoms

- Headaches
- Classic cause of **bitemporal hemianopsia**
- Compression of **optic chiasm**

JFW/Wikipedia

Hyperprolactinemia

- Women
  - Amenorrhea (lack of GnRH/LH/FSH)
  - Galactorrhea (prolactin)
- Men
  - "hypogonadotropic hypogonadism"
  - Decreased libido
  - Impotence
  - Infertility
  - Gynecomastia
  - Usually no galactorrhea (not enough breast tissue)

Prolactinoma

- Most common hormone secreting tumor
- **Headache, vision loss**
- Rarely seizures
- Women: amenorrhea, fractures (low bone density)
- Men: Loss of libido, impotence
- Diagnosis: serum prolactin; CNS imaging
- Treatment: Bromocriptine, cabergoline

Dopamine Antagonists

- Antipsychotics: Haloperidol, Risperidone
- Antiemetics: Metoclopramide
- Blockade of D2: ↑ **prolactin**
- Side Effects:
  - Amenorrhea
  - Breast engorgement
  - Galactorrhea
  - Sexual dysfunction
- Can also cause **Parkinsonian symptoms**

Hypopituitarism

- Caused by damage to anterior pituitary
  - Mass: Nonfunctional adenoma, craniopharyngioma
  - Ischemia, brain injury, hemorrhage
- ACTH deficiency
  - Low cortisol → **shock**
  - No loss of aldosterone → no salt wasting
  - Lack of hyperpigmentation (see in primary adrenal failure)
- TSH deficiency → hypothyroidism
- LH/FSH deficiency → hypogonadism

Craniopharyngioma

- Benign tumor
- Usually occurs in children 10-14 years old
- Symptoms from compression
  - Hypopituitarism
  - Headache, visual field defects
  - Behavioral change (frontal lobe dysfunction)
- Derived from remnants of Rathke's pouch

Empty Sella Syndrome

- Enlarged sella turcica partially filled with CSF
- Rarely can compress pituitary → hypopituitarism
- More common in **women** with **obesity, hypertension**

Radiation

- Some head and neck tumors treated with radiation
  - Brain tumors or nasopharyngeal carcinomas
- Some pituitary adenomas treated with radiation
- Can cause damage to hypothalamus or pituitary

Stevenfruitsmaak/Wikipedia

Pituitary Apoplexy

- **Sudden** hemorrhage into the pituitary gland
- Often occurs into **pre-existing adenoma**
- Risk factors for bleeding may be present (warfarin)
- Sudden onset severe headache
- Diplopia (pressure on oculomotor nerves)
- Hypopituitarism (**shock** from loss of cortisol)

Sheehan Syndrome

- Pituitary gland enlarged in pregnancy
- Vulnerable to infarction from hypovolemic shock
- Postpartum hemorrhage → hypopituitarism
- Can present as **shock after delivery**
- Also can see **failure to lactate**

Hypopituitarism
Treatment

- Hormone therapy
  - Corticosteroids
  - Thyroid hormone
  - Growth hormone
  - Estrogen/testosterone

Growth Hormone
Somatotropin

- Protein hormone
- Important for **linear (height) growth** in childhood
- Released in a pulsatile manner
- Between pulses levels may become undetectable

Growth Hormone
Somatotropin

- Many stimulants and suppressors
- Pituitary release stimulated by:
  - GHRH
  - Exercise
  - Sleep (very high just after onset of sleep)
- Released inhibited by:
  - Glucose
  - Somatostatin (released in response to IGF-1; GH)
  - IGF-1 (direct and indirect)

Growth Hormone Receptor

- Bind to a **membrane-bound** receptor
- Activates janus kinase 2 (**JAK2**) enzyme
  - Cytoplasmic tyrosine kinase
- Phosphorylates tyrosine residues
  - Within JAK 2 itself and on GH receptor
- Forms binding sites for many signaling molecules
- Alters gene expression

Growth Hormone

- **Liver** contains many growth hormone receptors
- GH → Liver → **IGF-1** secreted
  - Insulin-like growth factor 1/Somatomedin
  - Hormone that mediates many growth hormone effects
  - Can be **measured in serum** as indicator of GH function
- IGF-1 also produced in peripheral tissues
  - Paracrine effects on nearby sites

Growth Hormone
Direct Effects

- ↓ **glucose uptake by cells**
  - Anti-insulin
  - Will raise blood sugar ("Diabetogenic")
  - Peripheral tissues become insulin resistant
  - Hyperinsulinemia

Insulin

Glucagon
Cortisol
Epinephrine
Growth Hormone

Growth Hormone
Direct Effects

- Promotes lipolysis
  - Activates hormone sensitive lipase
- Production of IGF-1 from liver

Growth Hormone
IGF-1 Effects

- **Chondrocytes**
  - Increased linear growth
- Muscle
  - Lean muscle mass
- Organs
  - Increased organ size

Structure of a Long Bone

BruceBlaus/Wikipedia

Growth Hormone

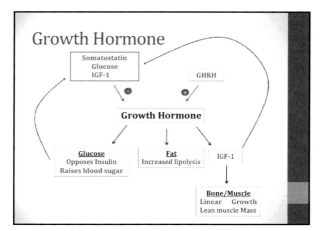

Growth Hormone Deficiency

- Children:
  - Failure to grow
- Adults
  - ↑ fat
  - ↓ lean body mass
  - Low energy

Growth Hormone Deficiency

- Most commonly from pituitary tumor
  - Mass effect
  - Consequence of surgery/radiation
- Treatment: Synthetic growth hormone
- Monitoring: **Serum IGF-1 level**

Growth Hormone Excess

- Most common cause is **somatotroph adenoma**
  - High GH and IGF-1
  - Low GHRH from hypothalamus (negative feedback)
  - High somatostatin (negative feedback)
  - May present with headache, vision loss
- Rare cause: GHRH secreting tumors
  - Hypothalamic tumors, carcinoid tumors, small-cell lung CA
  - GHRH level will be high

Growth Hormone Excess

- Children:
  - Excessive growth: **Gigantism**
  - Linear growth: Very tall child
- Adults: **Acromegaly**

Acromegaly

- Insidious onset
  - Average duration symptoms → diagnosis = 12 years
- **Enlarged jaw**
- Coarse facial features
  - Enlargement of nose, frontal bones

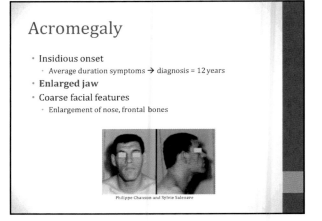

Philippe Chanson and Sylvie Salenave

Acromegaly

- Enlarged **hands and feet**
  - Classic sign: Increasing glove/shoe size
  - Rings that no longer fit

Acromegaly

- Insulin resistance → ↑ **insulin** → **diabetes**
  - Diabetes in 10-15% of patients
  - Abnormal glucose tolerance in 50% of patients

Glucagon
Cortisol
Epinephrine
Growth Hormone

Insulin

Acromegaly

- Visceral organs enlargement
  - Thyroid, heart, liver, lungs, kidneys, prostate
- Synovial tissue/cartilage enlargement
  - **Joint pain** in knees, ankles, hips, spine
  - Common presenting complaint is joint pain
- Cardiovascular disease
  - Hypertension, left ventricular hypertrophy, cardiomyopathy
  - **Mortality increased** in acromegaly due to CV disease

Growth Hormone Excess
Diagnosis

- **Serum IGF-1 concentration**
  - IGF-1 level is constant (contrast with GH)
- **Oral glucose tolerance testing**
  - Glucose should suppress growth hormone levels
  - Normal subjects: GH falls within two hours
  - Post glucose levels high
- CNS imaging (MRI)

Growth Hormone Excess
Treatment

- **Octreotide**
  - Analog of somatostatin
  - Suppresses release of growth hormone
- Also surgery, radiation
- Goal: **Lower IGF-1** to within reference range
- Bony abnormalities do not regress
- Joint symptoms often continue

MSH
Melanocyte Stimulating Hormone

- **Proopiomelanocortin**: Precursor of ACTH
- Also precursor of MSH (α/β/γ)
- MSH: Stimulates melanocytes to produce melanin
- Causes hyperpigmentation in **Cushing's disease**

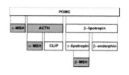

Oxytocin

- Produced in **paraventricular nuclei** of hypothalamus
- Causes **milk release** in response to suckling
  - Afferent fibers nipple → spinal cord
  - Triggers release oxytocin from posterior pituitary
  - Oxytocin triggers contraction of myoepithelial cells in breast

Oxytocin

- Also causes **contraction of uterus**
  - Oxytocin receptors upregulate in uterus near term
- Pitocin (synthetic oxytocin)
  - Induction of labor
  - Postpartum uterine bleeding

Somatostatin

- **Inhibits** release of many hormones
- Released by D cells throughout GI tract
- Also found in **nerves** throughout entire body
- Originally discovered in hypothalamus
- **Inhibits growth hormone release**
- Used therapeutically (Octreotide):
  - Acromegaly
  - Carcinoid syndrome
  - Glucagonoma/insulinoma
  - Upper GI bleeding (↓ splanchnic blood flow)

Parathyroid Glands

Jason Ryan, MD, MPH

Parathyroid Glands

- Four endocrine glands
- Formed by $3^{rd}/4^{th}$ pharyngeal pouch
- Located behind thyroid
- Secrete parathyroid hormone (PTH)
- Important for calcium, phosphate homeostasis

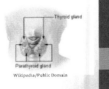

Wikipedia/Public Domain

Parathyroid Hormone

- Protein hormone
- Binds to cell **surface receptors in bone and kidney**
- Synthesized by **chief cells** of parathyroid gland

BruceBlaus/Wikipedia

Parathyroid Hormone Effects

- Net Effects:
  - $\uparrow [Ca^{2+}]$ plasma
  - $\downarrow [PO4^{3-}]$ plasma
  - $\uparrow [PO4^{3-}]$ urine
- Some effects due to direct action PTH
- Some due to activation of vitamin D (indirect)

Parathyroid Hormone

- Secreted in response to:
  - $\downarrow [Ca^{2+}]$ (major stimulus; fastest response)
  - $\uparrow$ plasma $[PO4^{3-}]$
  - $\downarrow 1,25-(OH)_2$ vitamin D
- Caclium activates calcium-sensing receptors (CaSRs)
  - $\downarrow$ PTH

Parathyroid Hormone
Magnesium

- High magnesium
  - $\downarrow$ PTH (same effect as calcium)
  - Magensium can activate CaSRs
- Low Mg
  - $\uparrow$ PTH release (same effect as calcium)
  - $\uparrow$ GI and renal magensium along with calcium

Parathyroid Hormone
Magnesium

- Very low Mg → inhibits PTH release
  - Some Mg required for normal CaSR function
  - Abnormal function → suppression of PTH release
  - Hypocalcemia often seen in severe hypomagenesemia

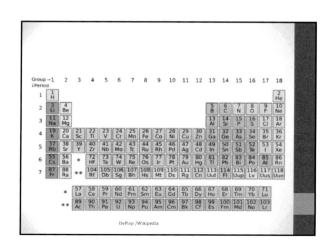

DePiep /Wikipedia

Qt Interval

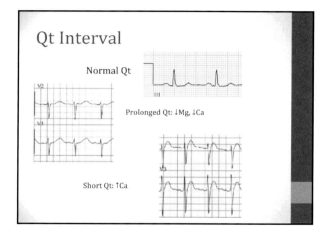

Normal Qt

Prolonged Qt: ↓Mg, ↓Ca

Short Qt: ↑Ca

Parathyroid Hormone Effects

- Kidney:
  - ↑ Ca^{2+} resorption (DCT)
  - ↓ $PO4^{3-}$ resorption (PCT)
  - ↑ 1,25-$(OH)_2$ vitamin D production
- GI:
  - ↑$Ca2+$ and $PO4^{3-}$ absorption (via vitamin D)
- Bone:
  - ↑$Ca2+$ and $PO4^{3-}$ resorption (direct and via vitamin D)

Parathyroid Hormone

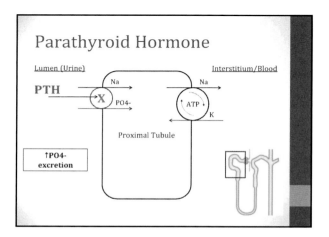

Lumen (Urine)   Interstitium/Blood

PTH

Na

X → PO4-

Na

ATP

K

Proximal Tubule

↑PO4- excretion

Vitamin D and the Kidney

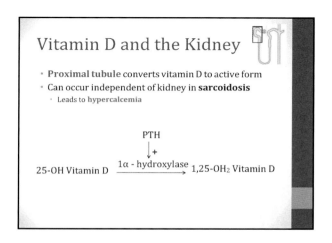

- **Proximal tubule** converts vitamin D to active form
- Can occur independent of kidney in **sarcoidosis**
  - Leads to **hypercalcemia**

PTH
↓ +

25-OH Vitamin D $\xrightarrow{1\alpha - \text{hydroxylase}}$ 1,25-OH_2 Vitamin D

Parathyroid Hormone

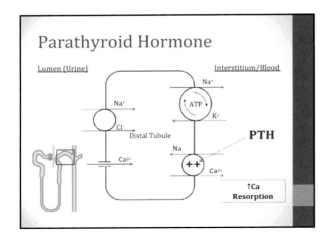

Lumen (Urine)　　　　　Interstitium/Blood

Distal Tubule

PTH

↑Ca
Resorption

Parathyroid Hormone

- Multiple effects on bone
- Stimulates bone **resorption and formation**
- Dominant effect varies with dosage/timing of administration of PTH to bone

Parathyroid Hormone

- Continuous administration of PTH
  - Bone resorption →↑ serum calcium
  - Important physiologically
- Low dose once daily bolus administration
  - Increased bone mass (bone formation)
  - **Teriparatide** used to treat osteoporosis

Parathyroid Hormone

- **Osteoblasts**
  - Bone forming cells
  - Contain PTH receptors
  - Can ↑ bone mass in response to PTH
- **Osteoclasts**
  - Bone resorbing cells
  - No PTH receptors
  - Activated indirectly by osteoblasts

Parathyroid Hormone

- **M-CSF**
  - Macrophage colony stimulating factor
  - Secreted by osteoblasts
- **RANK-L**
  - Receptor activating nuclear factor kβ ligand
  - Expressed on surface of osteoblasts
- Both produced by osteoblasts → activate osteoclasts

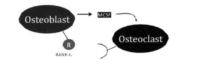

Types of Bone

- Cortical bone
  - Hard, outer layer of bone
  - ↓ in response to continuous PTH
- Trabecular bone
  - Spongy, inner layer of bone
  - ↑ in response to intermittent, low dose PTH

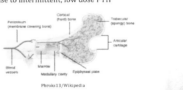

Pbroks13/Wikipedia

PTHrP
Parathyroid hormone-related protein

- Produced in many tissues
- Numerous normal effects
- Synthesized in large amounts by some **tumors**
  - Renal cell carcinoma
  - Squamous cell lung cancer
- Leads to **hypercalcemia** in malignancy

Hyperparathyroidism

- Primary (overactive glands)
- Secondary (hypocalcemia)
- Tertiary (seen in renal failure)

Primary Hyperparathyroidism

- Inappropriate secretion of PTH
- Not due to low calcium
- Commonly caused by **parathyroid adenoma**

Primary Hyperparathyroidism

- Causes **hypercalcemia**
  - ↑ renal reabsorption of Ca
  - ↑ vitamin D activation
  - ↑ bone resorption (loss of cortical bone)
- Phosphaturia

↑PTH ↑Ca

Primary Hyperparathyroidism

- Urinary calcium usually **high or normal**
- ↑ PTH → ↑ Ca urinary reabsorption → ↑ serum Ca
- ↑ serum Ca → ↑ urinary calcium

Primary Hyperparathyroidism
Symptoms

- "Stones, bones, groans, and psychiatric overtones"
  - Largely historical
  - Modern era, most patients diagnosed early
  - Often asymptomatic; diagnosis by routine blood work
  - **Recurrent kidney stones** is common presentation
  - Other signs/symptoms more often seen **malignancy**

Primary Hyperparathyroidism
Symptoms

- Stones (kidney)
  - High Ca in urine can cause stones
- Dehydration
  - Calcium blunts effects of ADH (nephrogenic DI)
  - Polyuria and polydipsia
  - Can lead to renal failure

Primary Hyperparathyroidism
Symptoms

- Bones (bone pain)
  - Adverse effects on bones of long-standing high PTH
- Groans (abdominal pain)
  - Constipation, anorexia, nausea
  - Increased stomach acid production (unclear mechanism)
  - Recurrent peptic ulcers
- Psychiatric overtones
  - Anxiety, altered mental status

Osteitis Fibrosa Cystica

- Classic bone disease of hyperparathyroidism
- Clinical features: Bone pain and fractures

Osteitis Fibrosa Cystica

- **Subperiosteal** bone resorption
  - Commonly seen in bones of fingers
  - Irregular or indented edges to bones
- **Brown tumors** (osteoclastoma)
  - Collections of giant osteoclasts in bone
  - Mixed with stromal cells and matrix proteins
  - Appear as black spaces in bone on x ray

Osteitis Fibrosa Cystica

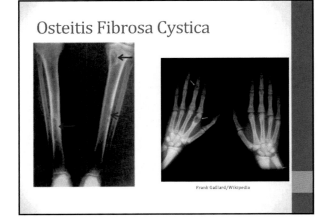

Frank Gaillard/Wikipedia

Primary Hyperparathyroidism
Treatment

- Parathyroidectomy
  - Removal of gland with adenoma
  - Pre-op nuclear imaging often done to identify location
- Risks of **recurrent laryngeal nerve** damage
  - May result in hoarseness
- Post-op **hypocalcemia**
  - Remaining parathyroid glands may be suppressed
  - Numbness or tingling in fingertips, toes, hands
  - If severe: twitching or cramping of muscles

2° Hyperparathyroidism

- Occurs in renal failure patients
- Chronically low serum calcium → ↑ PTH
- No symptoms of hypercalcemia
- Results in **renal osteodystrophy**
  - Bone pain (predominant symptom)
  - Fractures (weak bones 2° chronic high PTH levels)
  - If severe, untreated can lead to osteitis fibrosa cystica

↑PTH ↓Ca

3° Hyperparathyroidism

- Consequence of chronic renal failure
- Chronically low calcium → chronically ↑ PTH
- Parathyroid becomes autonomous
- VERY high PTH levels
- Calcium may become elevated
- Often requires parathyroidectomy

Calcium-Phosphate in Renal Failure

Sick Kidneys

↑**Phosphate**   ↓1,25-OH$_2$ Vitamin D

↓Ca from plasma   ↓Ca from gut

Hypocalcemia

↑PTH

FHH
Familial Hypocalciuric Hypercalcemia

- Rare, autosomal dominant disorder
- **Abnormal calcium sensing**
  - Abnormal calcium sensing receptors (CaSRs)
  - G-protein membrane receptors
  - Found in parathyroid and also kidneys
- Higher than normal set point for calcium
  - Normal PTH → ↑ calcium
- More renal resorption of calcium
  - Low urinary calcium

FHH
Familial Hypocalciuric Hypercalcemia

- Findings:
  - Usually normal PTH
  - Mildly elevated serum calcium
  - **Low urinary calcium** (key finding!)
- May looks like 1° hyperparathyroidism
- Real world distinction from 1° disease difficult
- Genetic testing available
- Usually does not require treatment

Hypoparathyroidism

- Inappropriately low PTH secretion
- Not due to hypercalcemia
- Causes **hypocalcemia**

↓PTH ↓Ca

Hypocalcemia
Signs/Symptoms

- Neuromuscular irritability
  - Nerves: **tingling** of fingers, toes, around mouth
  - Muscles: intermittent **spasms** (tetany)
- Tetany
  - Trousseau's sign: Hand spasm with BP cuff inflation
  - Chvostek's sign: Facial contraction with tapping on nerve
- Seizures

Hypoparathyroidism
Causes

- Surgical excision
  - Often accidental after thyroid or neck surgery
  - Key findings: post-op tingling, spasms
- Systemic diseases
  - Hemochromatosis (iron)
  - Wilson's (copper)
  - Metastatic cancer

APS-I
Autoimmune Polyendocrine Syndrome Type 1

- Rare autosomal recessive disorder
- Mutations of autoimmune regulator (AIRE) gene
  - AIRE also associated with chronic mucocutaneous candidiasis
- Triad:
  - Mucocutaneous candidiasis
  - Autoimmune hypoparathyroidism
  - Addison's disease

Thymic Aplasia
DiGeorge Syndrome

- Immunodeficiency syndrome
- Failure of 3rd/4th pharyngeal pouch to form
- Classic triad:
  - Loss of thymus (Loss of T-cells, recurrent infections)
  - Loss of parathyroid glands (hypocalcemia, tetany)
  - Congenital heart defects
- Presents in infancy/childhood with:
  - Hypocalcemia (hypoparathyroidism)
  - Recurrent infections
  - Congenital heart defects

Hypoparathyroidism
Treatment

- Calcium and calcitriol (vitamin D3)
- Recombinant human PTH available

Pseudohypoparathyroidism

- Group of disorders
- Kidney and bone unresponsiveness to PTH
  - **Abnormal PTH receptor** function
  - Many cases due to impaired G protein signaling
- Usually presents in childhood
- Hypocalcemia, hyperphosphatemia
- Elevated PTH (appropriate)

$$\uparrow \text{PTH} \quad \downarrow \text{Ca}$$

AHO
Albright's Hereditary Osteodystrophy

- Form of pseudohypoparathyroidism
- Autosomal dominant
- Hypocalcemia, hyperphosphatemia, ↑ PTH
- Collection of clinical features
  - Short stature
  - Shortened fourth and fifth metacarpals
  - Rounded facies
  - Mild mental retardation

Calcium and PTH

- 1st look at calcium: Low/High
- Next, look at PTH: Low/High
- Same direction = parathyroid problem
  - Both ↑: Hyperparathyroidism
  - Both ↓: Hypoparathyroidism
- Opposite direction
  - Normal response to calcium problem
  - Renal failure (low serum calcium – 2° hyperparathyroidism)
  - Renal losses (pseudohypoparathyroidism)

MEN Syndromes

Jason Ryan, MD, MPH

MEN Syndromes
Multiple Endocrine Neoplasia

- Group of rare genetic disorders
- **All autosomal dominant**
- Germline mutations in genes
- Lead to tumors in multiple endocrine glands
- MEN 1, 2A, 2B

MEN 1

- 3 P's
- Pituitary adenoma
- Parathyroid adenoma
- Pancreatic tumors

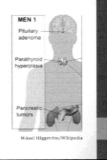

Mikael Häggström/Wikipedia

MEN 1

- Autosomal dominant
- Germline mutation of MEN1 gene (11q13)
  - Codes for the protein menin
  - Tumor suppressor
- Classic example of 2 hit hypothesis
  - Patients born with 1 abnormal MEN 1 gene
  - Second "hit" occurs in endocrine glands

MEN 1

- Parathyroid adenoma
  - Occurs in 94% of patients
  - First finding in ~90% of patients
  - Will present as hyperparathyroidism
  - Often detected when asymptomatic
  - May cause **recurrent kidney stones**

MEN 1

- Pituitary adenoma
  - Occurs in up to 70% of patients
  - Most commonly a prolactinoma
  - 2nd most common: GH secreting adenoma
- Pituitary adenomas not seen in other MEN syndromes
- **Pituitary disease = MEN 1**

MEN 1

- Pancreatic-duodenal neuroendocrine tumors
  - Most commonly a gastrinomas
  - Zollinger-Ellison syndrome: **multiple peptic ulcers**
  - Rarely insulinomas, gastrinomas, VIPomas

MEN 2A and 2B

- "Medullary" tumors
  - **Medullary** thyroid carcinoma
  - Pheochromocytoma (adrenal **medulla**)

Mikael Häggström/Wikipedia

MEN 2A and 2B

- MEN 2A
  - Medullary plus parathyroid
  - **No physical findings**
- MEN 2B
  - Medullary plus M's
  - Two key "phenotype" findings
  - Mucosal neuromas
  - Marfanoid appearance
  - Usually **no parathyroid involvement**

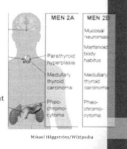

Mikael Häggström/Wikipedia

Medullary Carcinoma

- Cancer of parafollicular cells (C cells)
- Produces **calcitonin**
  - Lowers serum calcium
  - Normally minimal effect on calcium levels
  - With malignancy → **hypocalcemia**

MEN 2A and 2B

- MTC occurs earlier than sporadic cases
  - Sporadic: 60s
  - MEN: 30s
- ~100% risk of MTC
- Pheochromocytoma usually occurs after MTC

MEN 2B

- Same as 2A except:
  - Usually no parathyroid involvement
  - Two key physical findings
- #1: **Mucosal neuromas**
  - Lips, tongue
- #2: **Marfanoid** body habitus

MEN 2B Neuromas

- Benign growth of nerve tissue
- Often **lips and tongue**
- Sometimes intestinal neuromas

MEN 2B: Marfanoid

- **Tall**
- **Long wing span**
- High arched palate
- Skeletal deformations of spine:
  - Kyphoscoliosis: Curve to left/right
  - Lordosis: Curve forward
- No lens or aortic involvement (like Marfan's)

MEN 2A and 2B

- Autosomal dominant disorders
- Germline mutations in RET (chromosome 10)
- **Proto-oncogene**
- Codes for a **receptor tyrosine kinase**
- Important for cell growth/differentiation
- **Gain of function** mutations in MEN 2
  - Contrast with Hirschsprung disease of colon
  - Associated with loss of function mutations in RET

Thyroidectomy

- Often done **prophylactically** in MEN2 syndromes
- Usually at a young age (<5 years old)

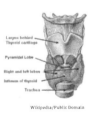

Wikipedia/Public Domain

MEN Syndromes

- Pituitary adenoma = MEN 1
- MTC or pheochromocytoma = MEN 2
- Parathyroid = MEN 1 or MEN 2A

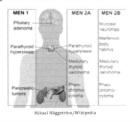

Mikael Häggström/Wikipedia

Signaling Pathways

Jason Ryan, MD, MPH

Hormone Effects

Hormone → Cell → Effects

Intracellular Hormones
Receptor in cytoplasm/nucleus

- Progesterone
- Estrogen
- Testosterone
- Cortisol
- Aldosterone
- Thyroid hormone

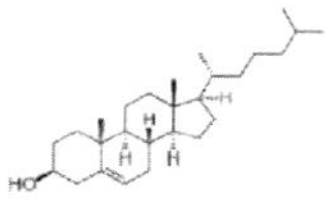

Cholesterol

Steroid Hormones

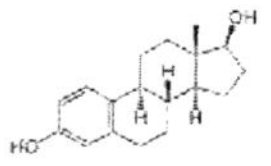

Estradiol
(17β-estradiol)

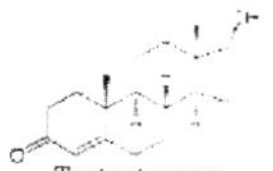

Testosterone

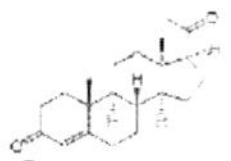

Progesterone

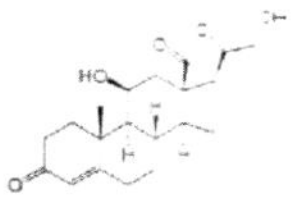

Aldosterone

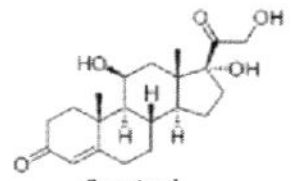

Cortisol

Thyroid Hormones

- Two hormones: T3 and T4
- Synthesized from tyrosine and iodine

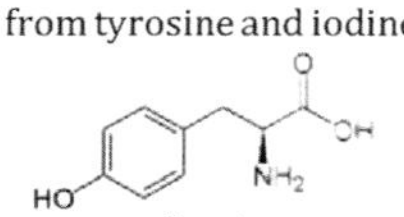

Tyrosine

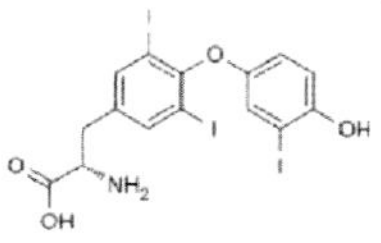

Triiodothyronine (T_3)

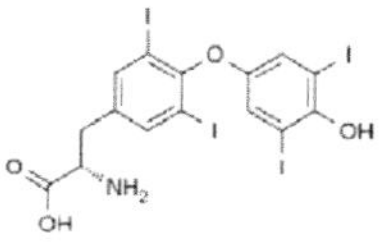

Thyroxine (T_4)

Intracellular Hormones

- All circulate **bound to a protein**
- Estrogen/testosterone: sex binding globulin (SBG)
- Thyroid hormone: thyroid binding globulin (TBG)
- Cortisol: corticosteroid-binding globulin (CBG)
  - Aldosterone
  - Progesterone

Extracellular Hormones

- Bind to **surface receptors**
- Use surface receptor to drive cellular changes
  - Tyrosine kinase
  - JAK/STAT
- Use **2ⁿᵈ messengers** to drive cellular changes
  - cAMP
  - cGMP
  - IP3

Receptor Tyrosine Kinase

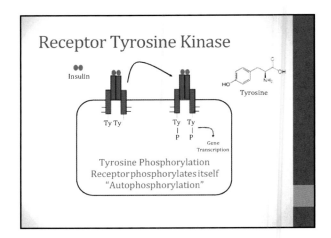

Tyrosine Phosphorylation
Receptor phosphorylates itself
"Autophosphorylation"

Receptor Tyrosine Kinase

- **Insulin**
- **Growth factors**
  - IGF-1 (insulin-like growth factor)
  - FGF (fibroblast growth factor)
  - PDGF (platelet-derived growth factor)
  - EGF (epidermal growth factor)

JAK/STAT

- Janus kinases (JAK)
  - Tyrosine kinase enzymes
- Signal Transducer and Activator of Transcription
  - STAT
  - Protein transcription factors
  - Activated by phosphorylation

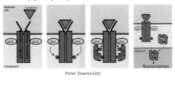

Peter Znamenkiy

JAK/STAT

- **Many cytokines**
  - IFN-γ, IL-2, IL-6
- **Bone marrow**
  - Erythropoietin
  - G-CSF (granulocyte-colony stimulating factor)
  - Thrombopoietin
- Others
  - Prolactin
  - Growth hormone

JAK2 Mutation

- Associated with myeloproliferative disorders
- Gene for cytoplasmic **tyrosine kinase**
- Mutation → ↑ tyrosine phosphorylation
- Progenitor cells: **hypersensitivity to cytokines**
- More growth; longer survival

Cyclic AMP

Hormone

Adenylyl Cyclase

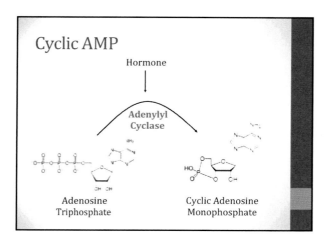

| Adenosine Triphosphate | Cyclic Adenosine Monophosphate |

G-Protein Linked Receptors

- Bind guanosine nucleotides (GDP, GTP)
- Transmit signals

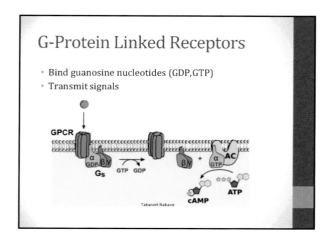

Cyclic AMP

- Hypothalamus
  - CRH, GHRH
- **Anterior pituitary hormones**
  - FSH, LH, ACTH, TSH
- **Parathyroid gland**
  - PTH, calcitonin
- Others
  - Glucagon
  - ADH (V2-receptor - water)
  - Histamine (H2-receptor – stomach acid)
  - hCG
  - MSH (melanocyte stimulating hormone)

Pituitary Hormones

- All have a **cAMP second messenger system**

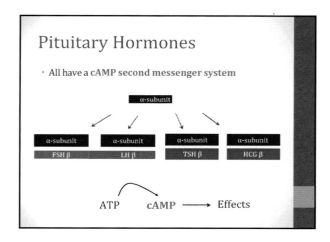

MSH

Melanocyte Stimulating Hormone

- Causes hyperpigmentation in **Cushing's disease**
- **Proopiomelanocortin**: Precursor of ACTH
- Also precursor of MSH ($\alpha/\beta/\gamma$)
- MSH: Stimulates melanocytes to produce melanin

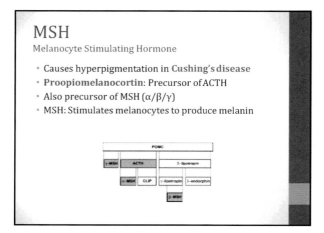

Cyclic GMP

Hormone

Guanylate Cyclase

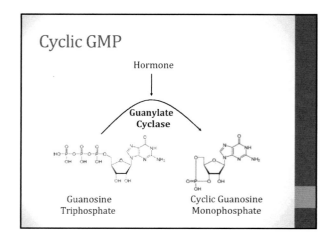

| Guanosine Triphosphate | Cyclic Guanosine Monophosphate |

Cyclic GMP

- **BNP/ANP**
  - Release by cardiac myocytes
  - Antagonize RAAS system
  - Both bind natriuretic peptide receptors (NPR)
  - Vasodilation/diuresis
- **Nitric oxide**
  - Endothelium-derived relaxing factor (EDRF)
  - Synthesized by endothelial cells
  - Activates cGMP → smooth muscle relaxation/vasodilation
- All are vasodilators

Inositol Triphosphate
IP3

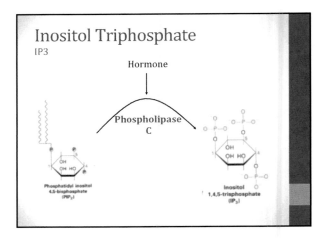

G-Protein Linked Receptors

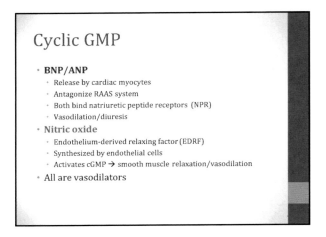

Inositol Triphosphate
IP3

- **Hypothalamus**
  - GnRH, TRH
- **Posterior Pituitary**
  - Oxytocin
  - ADH (**V1** receptor - vasoconstriction)
- **Others**
  - Histamine (**H1**-receptor – skin/lungs)
  - Angiotensin II
  - Gastrin

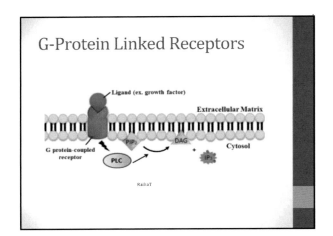

Hypothalamus

Hypothalamus	2nd Messenger
Corticotropin-releasing hormone (CRH)	cAMP
Thyrotropin-releasing hormone (TRH)	IP3
Gonadotropin-releasing hormone (GnRH)	IP3
Growth hormone–releasing hormone (GHRH)	cAMP

Anterior Pituitary

Hormone	2nd Messenger
Adrenocorticotropic hormone (ACTH)	cAMP
Thyroid-stimulating hormone (TSH)	cAMP
Luteinizing hormone (LH) Follicle-stimulating hormone (FSH)	cAMP
Growth hormone (GH)	JAK/STAT
Prolactin	JAK/STAT

Others

- IP3
  - ADH (V1 receptor)
  - Histamine (H1 receptor)
  - Gastrin
  - Angiotensin II
- cAMP
  - Histamine (H2 receptor)
  - AHD (V2 receptor)

Made in the USA
Coppell, TX
01 December 2019